C000021974

Where Doe

by
Anton Evans
and
Louise van Wingerden

Cover illustration by
Lucy Markes (Frog Prints)

Published by Twynham Press
Paperback 1st edition

ISBN 978-095669376-1

Dedications

This book is dedicated to my first GP, Dr Cantlie, and also to the GPs and nurses at the Barn Surgery, Purewell. I would also like to thank Great Ormond Street Hospital and its Tadworth Court Country Branch for the care they gave me. I will never forget the kindness that I received there.

Many thanks also to Southampton General Hospital, Alton Hospital, Poole Hospital, the Royal Bournemouth Hospital and Christchurch Hospital for their help and treatment over the years – and also to Dorset Adult Services.

I would like to acknowledge my great debt to Moore Bros. Surgical Shoes, without whose help over the years I would have been a lot less mobile.

I would also like to thank Somerford Infants and Junior School, Twynham Comprehensive and the Bournemouth and Poole College of Art.

Finally, I must express my everlasting gratitude to my Mum and Dad and my big sister Julie. You are the heroes of my story, and I love you dearly.

CONTENTS

FOREWORD by Louise van Wingerden

I was introduced to Anton Evans in early 2012. A friend, Rosie Groves, asked whether I would consider ghost-writing a book for her husband's old school friend. Rosie told me that this chap had been born severely disabled but nonetheless had built an independent and successful life for himself and gone on to help many others with his charity work and fund raising. Indeed, all the proceeds from the sale of this book will be donated to two children's charities, Great Ormond Street Hospital and The Children's Trust. I hope you enjoy reading it as much as I have enjoyed helping Anton to write it.

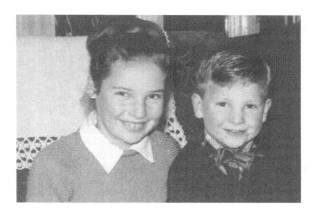

Julie (sister) and Anton, 1960's

1

Chapter One
The Early Years

I was born at two minutes before midnight on the 17th October, 1958 at my grandparents' house at Purewell, in Christchurch, Hampshire. It was an impressive building – Ashtree House, which at that time was a riding school.

For the first two years of my life I stayed at Ashtree House with my Mum and Dad, Jim and June Evans, my older sister Julie and our grandparents. We had a home of our own, but my Nanny was ill and so we stayed at Ashtree so that Mum could help to look after her.

I was a bonny baby, weighing exactly seven and a half pounds and apparently physically healthy. My Mum still remembers how, when I was just one year old, I used to sit in my high chair and refuse to eat my food.

'I'm not having any of that' I would say to myself, and instead of using my spoon and fork to manoeuvre the food into my mouth I would use them to flick it all around the room. Kitchen walls, table and chairs, all would be satisfyingly splattered with baby food at breakfast, lunch and dinner times.

I had a blue plastic cup with a built-in plastic straw and according to Mum what I liked to do best, as I sat marooned in my high chair, was to drink milk from this cup, blowing bubbles and at the same time chewing the plastic straw with my new front teeth. I was a proper mucky pup, she says.

Everything seemed normal enough, but there was something darker lurking in the background of this happy family picture; a growing sense of concern. My

Mum was patiently trying to move me on to the next stage of development; trying to teach me to stand up and walk, but I kept sitting down and crawling along the floor instead. As I crawled I cried, as if in pain.

Mum and Dad persevered, and eventually things improved slightly. I started to walk, just a few steps at a time. Progress was slow though, and eventually Mum commandeered Julie, who was four and a half years older, to keep an eye on me while she got on with the housework.

As time went on though, it became apparent that I was very small for my age. I also didn't seem to make progress in my ability to move. My legs hurt all the time, and even when I managed to walk a few steps I would scream with the pain. Even when Mum pushed me along in the pushchair I would cry at every bump we encountered in the pavement. Something was up, but nobody knew quite what, and all the adults in my life were gradually becoming more concerned.

It was early in 1964, and I was five years old, when my parents took me to see our local GP, Dr Cantlie. He immediately wrote a referral for me to see a specialist. Things happened fast from that point – I was given an appointment at the Great Ormond Street Hospital for Sick Children in the City of London, just a few weeks later. I was going to see an orthopaedic surgeon specialist, a Mr Lloyd Roberts.

When the day of the appointment dawned, I remember that my parents and I had to get up very early in the morning to catch an express steam train. We were due to travel from Christchurch railway station to Waterloo station in London.

I was excited at the prospect of a trip to London, but as the train drew up in front of us at the station I stood petrified with fear. This train was a massive black beast, and the steam rushing out from its wheels and engine was overwhelmingly loud. I cheered up when the train driver and fireman both smiled and waved at me. Mum, Dad and I were privileged – first class seats had been reserved for us by the National Health Service. So we enjoyed a leisurely walk along the platform to our designated seats, while all around us others rushed and clamoured, jostling to get the best positions in the ordinary carriages.

And so the journey to London began. I was fascinated, and yet intimidated, by the group of identical-looking bowler-hatted businessmen who shared our carriage. They looked to me like the little men on the TV adverts for self-raising flour – and there they sat, all lined up, straight-faced and impenetrable reading their newspapers, while I was squeezed between them clutching my Batman comic.

At first I was riveted by the new experience, but before long it became tedious - this journey seemed to be going on and on. Eventually, things seemed to be reaching a climax - the train was gathering speed, crossing lines that linked with other trains travelling simultaneously. It felt to me as though we were going to come right off our track.

I knew that we were close to London now, and I could see that this place was very different to the quiet Hampshire town that I had travelled from (incidentally, the County borders have changed since I was a child and Christchurch is now in Dorset). There were tall flats, with washing hanging off the balconies, and children playing on the rooftops. There was a terrible smog over the city – at times I could hardly see through the thick glass of the train window, and this was in the daylight! London seemed a strange sort of a place to me.

But now we had arrived at Waterloo station, and at last we could disembark from our train. It looked as if there were thousands of people milling around in this small space, and I wondered where on earth all these people could be going.

Mum gripped my hand very tightly, stooping down to my level to tell me she was hanging on to me in case I got lost in the crowds. 'I need to wee!' I wailed, so she handed me to my father, who took me through a small tunnel to some loos. There were lots of men standing in line there. Trying to make sense of what was happening, I realised to my surprise that the Station toilets doubled as a Gentlemen's hairdressing shop. What a strange new world this was.

We made our way back to Mum, and then the three of us walked together to the station exit. Here I was also taken aback - I had never seen so many uniformly sized and coloured cars waiting in line in my whole life. The businessmen in their bowler hats were shouting, 'Taxi, Taxi!' and so my Dad shouted out too, 'Taxi!' and in seconds a black cab materialised before us like magic.

'Where do you want to go to, Guv'nor?' the driver asked. Dad said, 'Could you take us to the Great Ormond Street Hospital for Sick Children please?' So the taxi driver navigated us through London city, and it was a massive place, bigger than I had ever imagined.

Eventually we arrived at Great Ormond Street Hospital. I knew by now that this journey was all about me, but I was still sketchy about the details, and I felt very scared as we made our way through the grand entrance to the reception desk and announced ourselves. A very kind lady helped us sign in and showed us to the waiting room.

I was familiar by now with our local hospital and clinics, and there were no toys in any of them. In this room, by contrast, toys littered the floor and no-one seemed to mind. There were rocking horses, teddy bears six feet tall... it was a toy emporium, a wonderland.

I waited with Mum and Dad, and we watched as a constant stream of children arrived to see the specialist. These children were mostly in wheelchairs, and I could see that they were all different shapes and sizes. Each of them was unique, and totally unlike any person or child that I had met before. It was only then, in the waiting room of the orthopaedic specialist at Great Ormond Street Hospital for Sick Children, that I realised that I was one of these special children.

I had a very short right leg, small fingers, small feet and a slightly twisted rib cage. I had a bent back and a stiff neck, although my face, nose, mouth and eyes were all normal. I had known for some time that I was different from my friends, but until that point I had honestly not realised that I was disabled.

It was a distressing sight. I could see that my Mum and Dad were watching too, holding back tears while trying not to stare at these many children, all suffering from different illnesses and disabilities. A lot of parents looked stressed and worried, as I suppose was natural given the difficulty of their positions and the uncertainty of their futures.

Eventually a nurse called out my name and I was ushered in to see the specialist, Mr Lloyd Roberts. I put on my best brave face, and I regarded him carefully as he talked. He looked like a professor, with heavy black-framed glasses that perched precariously on the tip of his nose.

I was subjected to a lot of tests and X-rays. These procedures took many hours, but eventually we were ushered back in to see the consultant, who announced that my diagnosis was Morquio's Syndrome. We were told that this was a rare genetic disorder, and that sufferers could have a variety of symptoms, including heart and joint problems and restricted growth. Although there was no cure, the specialist assured my parents that with care I could lead a happy life.

With those few words, the way I understood my whole world had changed.

Chapter Two
Growing Up

Later that year, Mum Dad and I went on another trip to Great Ormond Street. This time we went to see the surgical shoemaker, whose task it was to design me some new footwear. The specialist had instructed him to make my right shoe an inch and a half higher than the left because that was how far shorter the leg measured on that side. The shoemaker informed us that the shoes would be handmade by Prior and Howard, a company which manufactures specialist shoes and limbs for Great Ormond Street and many other British hospitals. It would take the shoemaker roughly three weeks to have the shoes ready. Then, he said, they would be posted to us.

I looked forward to getting my new shoes, and reluctantly resigned myself to the three weeks' wait. The day they arrived was a red letter day. There was the parcel, on the kitchen table. I set to immediately, ripping off the paper in my eagerness to get to my new footwear. But as the shoes finally stood unwrapped we all stared at them in shock. The four of us had all fallen silent. The left shoe was passable, but the right one was like something out of a horror movie. It looked just like Herman Munster's shoes – the ones he wore in the 1960's children's television programme.

The shoe was a big heavy solid box coloured jet black, with black shoelaces. I felt myself engulfed by panic and choked with fear and I ran crying into the living room. I would look like a monster if I wore those shoes. There was no way I could ever wear them in the presence of my friends at Somerford Infants School. No way, ever.

And it was not just the reaction of my friends I feared - I could see that everyone I knew would laugh and stare and mock me if I was to wear these shoes. Every child and every adult who ever saw me would make fun of me. I hated those shoes.

Dad disappeared then, and he was gone for over an hour. When he came back he presented me with a Hornby train set. He had brought a surprise parcel for Julie too – because although she had not suffered any trauma, Mum and Dad were always keen to make sure that both of us were treated equally at all times.

Eventually, with the help of my new train set, I managed to calm down. Mum persuaded me to try the shoes on, and now I felt that I looked like Herman Munster and even walked like him. I could hardly believe that a few hours ago I had really thought that these shoes would make my life better.

Somehow, with the help and reassurance of my family, I realised that I just had to get on with it. I did wear the shoes to school the next morning, sure that I would be an instant social outcast, but to my amazement my school friends were glad to see me as usual and greeted me as if nothing was amiss.

During the course of the morning a few children did ask, 'Why are you wearing a funny built up shoe?' but by then I had developed a plan. I replied to each of them the same, 'I keep my pocket money in it' and the notion of shillings and notes rattling around in my shoes seemed to distract them successfully, because nothing else was said.

I liked my Infants School, and I did well there. One day I wrote a story about my Dad, who was a part-time fireman for the Hampshire Fire Brigade. I painted a picture of him to go with the story. He had a big black helmet, a silver buttoned thick black fireman's jacket, black fireproof trousers and an axe fitted onto his belt.

By now we no longer stayed at Ashtree House, but were back living in our own home nearby. We lived in a small detached house on the Somerford estate. What I liked best about it was that my Dad had a fire bell fitted at home, connected to the telephone line, and when this rang it meant that Dad was being called out to a fire.

I found it all terribly exciting. One evening as we were waiting for Coronation Street to come onto the TV, the fire bell rang. Dad dashed out of the lounge and outside to his Morris Minor Estate, and then drove at full pelt to Christchurch Fire Station. We found out later that Fawley Oil Refinery, owned by Esso, had been alight. My Dad, along with many other firemen and reserves from stations along the South Coast, had been called out, all risking their lives in order to deal with the explosion.

It was not the first or the last time. Fawley Refinery had many outbreaks of fire each year, and sometimes we didn't see Dad for days after a major incident. It must have been a huge worry to my Mum, but to me it was a great source of drama and entertainment.

My Dad was not just a part-time fireman though. He was a plumber too, and a central heating engineer. He worked hard, and my mother was busy too. She helped my grandparents out at their nearby home, Ashtree House. Ashtree was a large farmhouse, with ten acres of land. My Nanny used half an acre to grow many different varieties of daffodil and my Mum helped her to sell these daffodils, and chicken eggs too, to local customers.

Grandad also had a fruit and vegetable wholesale business in Bournemouth. He supplied local hotels and schools, including my own school. I often saw Grandad hauling large sacks of potatoes into school, handing them over to the cooks who prepared our meals.

Around that time, my grandparents embarked on a new business enterprise, to turn Ashtree House into a riding school. Mum and her brother, my Uncle Matt, were heavily involved in the new riding school. Grandad decided to refurbish the farmhouse - he painted the outside white, and fixed yellow wooden shutters to the sides of the windows. He then got a sign made up to advertise the riding school, and put it in the front garden, facing the main road.

Grandad called the new business Ashtree Riding School. He built fifteen stables there, along with two tack rooms, a large hay barn and several feed rooms. There were paddocks too, with floodlights, and my grandparents equipped the school with many horses and ponies.

My Grandad employed people to run the school and installed his top BHS riding instructor in a house he bought across the road from the farmhouse. My Mum went out with Grandad delivering business cards to advertise Ashtree Riding School to all the hotels in Bournemouth. We were an industrious family.

Grandad soon expanded the business. He was full of ideas. He started Day Treks in the New Forest. He set up a Pony Club. He organised Gymkhanas and camping riding holidays.

The Riding School was great fun, and I took part in various activities there. I liked to dress up, pretending to be a cowboy, riding my Nanny's Shetland pony, Bambi. I once took part in a fancy dress competition on horseback at Ashtree Riding School in my favourite outfit. I still remember the joy and the pain of that day – my condition was bad, and I was trying not to cry out in agony each time that Bambi moved. I wouldn't give up though, and managed to hang on until the end, with Dad supporting me on the horse. I came second and won a rosette.

Success must have gone to my head, because later in the same year I took part in another fancy dress competition at Ashtree, dressing up as a horseradish made out of crepe paper. This time I rode 'Coco' – a pony named after the famous English circus clown. I sat proudly upon my charger, but as the judges approached the riders, rain began to fall, first in light drops but soon after in a solid sheet. The colours from my costume dripped into my eyes and down my face. I couldn't see, and I was scared, but I sat firm. I was hoping for another rosette.

But it was not to be. Just as the judges reached me, the horse bolted and went flying off into the next paddock, with me clinging on for dear life. My crepe paper outfit was sodden and disintegrating, and I was covered from head to foot in horseradish-coloured dye. Everybody watching was hysterical with laughter at the spectacle. Never mind Coco the horse – I was the attraction here and I felt like Coco the Clown myself!

The years passed. In September 1966, when I was seven years old, I moved up from Somerford Infants to Somerford Junior School. Mr Hackett, my new headmaster, had heavy black eyebrows and a receding hairline. He always wore a grey suit. His voice was curiously high pitched, and so it stood in stark contrast to his severe demeanour. Mrs Hackett, his wife, was the headmistress and was in charge of the girls in the school.

The day I started at the Juniors I knew it was the beginning of a new era. I wore black shorts and a grey shirt, a black and white striped tie, grey socks and a black school cap with the school logo on it. The outfit was completed by my special black surgical shoes.

It was a large school, and every day I would come across new children that I had never seen before. I was still embarrassed by the horrible big black built up shoe, and this time my fears were realised from the start. In my old school everybody had known me and they had all been kind, but here all the children seemed to be looking sideways at me and laughing.

The questions came thick and fast.

'Why are you so small?'

'Why are you wearing that funny built-up shoe?'

And the worst of all, 'Peg leg! Peg leg!'

I needn't have worried though, because my friends from the Infant School soon stood up for me. They spread the word about my disability. 'Antony was born with a serious condition called Morquio's Syndrome' they said. 'And how would you like it if you were born like that, and somebody called you names and laughed at you because of it?'

The bullies were soon silenced, and I had learned something too – the importance of speaking up in self-defence. Often, I realised, cruelty has its roots in ignorance and with understanding comes respect.

After a few weeks had passed, I relaxed and started to enjoy school more. I was particularly interested in music, and had taught myself to play the piano a little. One of my friends told the music teacher, Mrs Tickner, about this and she called me into the music room and asked me to play to her.

I did as she asked, and when I looked up at the end I was surprised to see that she had tears in her eyes. 'You played so beautifully' she said. 'Did you make that up yourself?'

'No' I said, 'It is called 'Les Petites Enfants' which means 'Little Children'. I heard it on a French radio station and I copied it'. I told her that I had also picked up some of the French language, and she was very impressed.

I liked to read Ladybird books, particularly the ones about the Police Service, Fire Brigade and Hospitals. I had to choose one of these books to read to my English teacher, in front of the whole class. So I chose the Fire Brigade book, because my Dad was a fireman and I was proud of that.

The book had pictures to illustrate the story, and after I had read my book to the class I was told to copy a picture from the book and to write my own story about it. I already liked writing, but that was the moment when I realised for the first time that I was much better at drawing than most of the other children.

We all handed our work in to the teacher. We all waited as she marked it, sitting at her desk in front of us. When she suddenly called out, 'Antony Evans, come here at once!' I was convinced that I had done something wrong, and I made my way to her side tentatively.

She smiled at me warmly. 'Well done little man,' she said. 'You have done some brilliant work today, and you get a Gold Star.'

I was so happy and buoyed up. I couldn't wait to get home and tell my Mum and Dad about my success with the story and the picture. Julie had always done very well at school, and I felt that I was destined to follow in her footsteps.

At the weekends, school was out. I mostly stayed at home and watched TV (in black and white because that was all we had) or played with my toys. I liked Lesney Matchbox cars and every weekend would start with a Friday evening visit to the toy shop in Christchurch where I would buy another car for my collection. I got two shillings and sixpence of pocket money each week, and it was all spent on toys.

After the toy shop Mum, Dad and I would head to the local supermarket, Fine Fare, where we bought the food for the coming week. One Friday, to my delight, Mum let me push the trolley. I was in my element. It was all going well. But then as Mum turned around sharply to take a box of cereal from a high shelf, I swung the trolley around in her wake, without first checking to see what was behind me.

With a mighty crash, bang and wallop my trolley collided with a tall stack of tins of peas. What seemed like hundreds of tins of peas went flying all over the shop. Mum was pink with embarrassment and in my confusion I hid around the counter as all eyes searched for the cause of the commotion.

To my relief the manager of the shop burst out laughing. 'Don't worry, young man,' he said to me. 'I knew I should not have put those peas in that particular place'. He seemed unable to contain his laughter. Mentally, I immediately cast myself starring alongside Sid James in the Carry On film of 'Crash, Bang, Wallop at Fine Fare Supermarket'.

As a treat, sometimes on a Saturday afternoon Mum would take Julie and I to the Regent Cinema in Christchurch to watch a Disney film. One memorable day we went to see Doctor Who and the Daleks. I still remember it now – it was called Invitation Earth, and it starred Peter Cushing, Roberta Tovey, Jennie Linden and Roy Castle.

I had been so looking forward to this film. I waited eagerly in the cinema next to my Mum and my sister, counting the moments until 3pm when the film was due to begin. It was brilliant, all I had hoped for and more. A thrilling, action-packed adventure. I hardly noticed the time passing.

Mum did, though. The film was still half an hour from its climax when she suddenly announced that Julie had a ballet lesson starting shortly up the road. We had to leave now.

I couldn't bear it. I was expected to leave the film, at this stage, just to take Julie to her dance lesson! I called my sister every name I could think of, culminating in the worst insult my imagination could conjure, 'I hope you turn into a frog'. Unfortunately she didn't, so we had to leave the cinema and I never got to see what happened to Doctor Who or to the Daleks. I was extremely disgruntled.

We travelled home on the bus after Julie's lesson, and let ourselves in through the front door. My Dad, innocent as to what had happened, called out to me from upstairs, 'Did you enjoy your Dr Who film, Antony?'

'No, Dad,' I fired back. 'I have just been Exterminated by Julie's ballet lesson'.

Around that time, Mum and Dad decided that Julie and I should attend Sunday School at the local church. I was not impressed with the idea from the start. 'Boring,' I said to myself at the prospect, as any seven year old boy would have done. Of course, I had no choice, and so we found ourselves at the Baptist Church near Christchurch town centre every Sunday morning at 9am sharp. I rapidly discovered that Sunday School was every bit as tedious as I had predicted.

I liked the Church itself well enough. It was a quirky little building, full of interesting dark nooks and crannies. I deeply resented having to sit through services though, and especially having to put a threepenny piece in the collection bag every week.

What a waste, I thought. And so I devised a plan. My hands were tiny, and I found that for once this gave me an advantage. I could easily fit my whole hand into the velvet collection bag, gripping my coin. Then I would pretend to drop the coin in, but actually just remove my hand from the bag neatly, fist still tightly closed around my thruppenny bit. Ha! Fooled them!

I didn't fool Julie, though. She was getting quite religious at that time, and when she saw what I was up to she did her best to put the fear of God into me. 'If you keep doing that,' she hissed at me one Sunday, 'Your hands will get even smaller'.

I took no notice of my sister. Julie wouldn't be around much longer anyway, as she had hatched some sort of a plan herself, to go off and become a nun or a missionary somewhere. Mum and Dad were none too pleased about their teenage daughter's religious zeal, but I thought it was rather a good idea.

Unfortunately (in my opinion) Julie changed her mind after attending one church meeting too many. She came home one evening having decided that she had been quite put off religion by all the politics and bickering she had witnessed. Mum and Dad heaved a sigh of relief, and I heaved the sigh of a long-suffering younger brother who was to be further burdened with the presence of his bossy teenage sister.

One cold winter morning I was hanging about waiting for a lift to Sunday School. I didn't mind the thought of a lift, but I was astonished when it arrived. An old man pulled up outside our house on his motor bike. His wife, an old lady, was sitting in the sidecar. She gestured to me. 'Get in, boy!' she insisted as I stared in dismay.

There was no free space that I could see.

Obediently though, I clambered somehow into the old sidecar, between the old lady's legs, almost smothered by her long blue silk dress. It was very cramped in there; neither of us could move much and I could hardly breathe. The old man put on his goggles, to protect his eyes from the wind, and off we went with a mighty roar as the engine started up.

It was not a smooth journey, to say the least. The sidecar was shaking, rattling and rolling all over the place, and vibrating heavily. I was petrified with fear. Then, just as we approached the church, the old man leaned to turn his motorbike right, and the old lady and I failed to take the turn alongside him. The sidecar had become detached from the bike, and so instead we went rolling down the road for several yards. Meanwhile, somehow the sidecar had inverted and so the pair of us were upside down to boot.

As we eventually came to a halt, I tried to extract myself from the vehicle. To my immense embarrassment though, I was wedged in, with my face squashed on the old lady's big boobs, right against the side car window, gazing out at the small crowd of shocked bystanders who seemed to have materialised from nowhere.

It felt like minutes, but was probably only seconds before I managed to kick the side door open with my built up shoe (for once that thing had come in useful). Between them the assembled group then pulled the two of us out of the infernal contraption. The old lady and I were both unharmed.

Once again I escaped from shameful reality by

envisaging myself as the star of a movie. I bowed to the crowds before me on the imaginary red carpet.

James Bond, at your service. Shaken, but not stirred.

Chapter Three
Broken Shoes, Scotland & the Beautiful Game

Around that time I encountered serious problems with my surgical shoes. The leather was breaking away from the soles, and I could not walk in them safely. When Mum rang the shoemaker at Great Ormond Street she was told that it would take several weeks to make a new pair.

So my life was put on hold. I was housebound. At first this was a novelty. I was not short of entertainment, because although there was no television in the daytimes back then, there always seemed to be something happening in the street outside our front windows.

The baker came by most days, delivering fresh bread in baskets. The milkman clattered up and down in his horse and trap. The yellow open air lorry that sold Corona soft drinks rattled past noisily, followed by the two wheeled cart pushed along by the man who called out, 'Rag and Bone!' Ice cream vans, emblazoned with the logos of Toni Bell, Walls or Mr Whippy, played the tunes that all the neighbourhood children knew so well. The window cleaner would make a regular appearance, ladders fixed to his push bike and trailer.

There was another man with a dynamo attached to his bicycle wheel. He would set his bicycle upside down on the pavement, and use the contraption to sharpen people's garden shears and knives there at the side of the road as the wheel spun. I saw travellers who sold flowers door to door. Ladies promoting new household products such as Fairy Liquid to wash the dishes. The coal man, who brought the coal that heated our house. The chimney sweep, the Avon lady, the man who collected the shillings each week from our electricity meter. The rich tapestry of life was played out along our street every day, and it provided a good diversion while I was stuck at home without any shoes.

The novelty soon paled though. I had been doing well at school and I was eager to learn. I was already starting to feel frustrated by the pain that made it difficult for me to concentrate as well as I would have liked. Now I was denied the opportunity to attend at all, and I was sure that I would soon fall behind and find it hard to catch up.

It wasn't all bad. One morning a lady knocked at the door. She was promoting a new sort of food – something I had never seen before – a potato crisp. These were the Golden Wonder variety – they had a cartoon of a Scotsman on the packet. They were delicious, as I ascertained from the free sample she gave me to try. She said they came in different flavours, and I couldn't wait to taste the others.

Two weeks came and went, and I was still at home. The whole family was becoming frustrated by the wait for my shoes now. Mum rang up Great Ormond Street again, only to hear that there was a delay because they were waiting for the new black leather to arrive. 'It could take another week or more to get your son's shoes made, I'm afraid'.

I missed my friends most of all. One day in the late afternoon a bunch of them dropped by to see me. By then the Headteacher, Mr Hackett, had become notorious for the liberal use he made of his long thin cane, and I was treated to the chilling tales of his latest victims. Being disabled, of course, I was safe from the dreaded cane, and I was never scared of the Headteacher, although others were. (Mr Hackett had doted on my sister Julie, who had left the Junior School just as I arrived, and he always greeted me with enthusiasm, as though I was a long lost friend. I didn't mind this, although I was annoyed that he always addressed me as Tony).

Anyway, the days were dragging on and still the new shoes had not arrived. I indulged myself with television – many of these programmes were an education in themselves, and sometimes I was allowed to stay up late to watch them. I sucked it all up, although increasingly I just wanted to get away from all this fantasy, back to my real life. But I was stuck indoors and that was all there was to it.

It was my Uncle Matt, Mum's brother, who came to my rescue. He phoned up from Ashtree House one day, and spoke to my Mum. 'I have to go to Scotland, to Ayr, to collect three horses, tomorrow morning. I was wondering whether Antony would like to come along for the trip?'

I was close to my Mum, listening by the receiver, and I didn't wait for her to relay my Uncle's message. 'Yes, please!' I shouted as loudly as I could in the direction of the phone.

We left at six o'clock the next morning. It was a two day trip, so Matt loaded up the Landrover with camping beds and enough food and drink to last the three of us (he'd brought along another man to share the driving). We climbed into the vehicle. 'Bye then!' I called to my parents.

'Bye!' they called back. 'Bye Matt! Oh – and if Antony talks too much, just stop his mouth with the black tape we bought to patch his shoes up!' And we were off.

I waved goodbye to Mum and Dad out of the back of the Landrover, poking out my tongue out at them for good measure. Me – talk too much? The cheek!

The journey began well. We were on the motorway, making good time. But then as Uncle Matt moved the Land Rover out to the middle lane to overtake a lorry, the bonnet flew up, landing loudly, flat and tight against the front of the windscreen. Matt was travelling at full speed, and now suddenly he couldn't see an inch of the road, which was crammed with other vehicles. We braced ourselves for the collision.

I was really scared, but fortunately my uncle stayed calm. I watched in wonder as he wound down the driver's side window and leaned out of it to see the road, using his left hand to steer. Luckily the lorry driver had seen what was happening and drove slowly to block the inside lane so that we could glide over to the hard shoulder. We pulled over, all of us dizzy with relief.

The black shoe tape did come in useful then, to securely fasten down the Land Rover bonnet. We continued on our journey, still shaken by our narrow escape from disaster. I suddenly realised that something else was awry. It had started to rain outside – but surely the rain should not be falling inside our vehicle? 'Um,' Uncle Matt, 'I said. 'This Landrover is leaking like a sieve'.

It was indeed, and so we stopped at a nearby service station and deployed more of the black shoe tape to stop the rain coming in through the roof. After quick refreshments and refuelling we started off again, and at 10pm we finally reached the Scottish border.

We were at what was known as a 'Checkpoint Charlie' - the military police were stopping all the vehicles and checking them for bombs on their undersides, because there had been problems in the area with the IRA. There was a long delay, but eventually we were told that we could carry on our way.

By now, though, we'd all had enough. Matt stopped in the nearest layby. We didn't even unpack the camp beds. I slept in the back of the Land Rover, tucked inside the big spare tyre, Uncle Matt slept in the box trailer we'd brought to collect the horses, and the other driver slept across the two front seats of the Land Rover, his face wedged onto the steering wheel.

It was freezing that night. I lay curled in my tyre staring at the car roof, exhausted, overwrought and homesick. I must have managed to get some sleep eventually, because at six o'clock the next morning Uncle Matt woke me, and then we were all confronted with our next problem.

We were surrounded by thick fog and had no clue where we were. Luckily, beside us was a lorry whose driver had also obviously slept the night in the layby. My uncle asked him the way to Ayr.

'You're facing the wrong way for Ayr,' smiled the man. 'It's behind you, about fifty miles back. But be very careful driving down the mountain, you could easily slide and crash. Good luck'.

We'd arrived in the dark, and only saw now what a precarious position we were in, perched high on the side of a mountain with a steep drop at the side of the road. Uncle Matt was in a bad mood. He looked over at the other driver. 'Help,' he growled.

It took more than an hour for us to crawl slowly back down the mountain. At least we were heading the right way now, and several hours later we finally reached our destination. We were greeted by an enormous Scotsman who, to my amusement, looked and spoke like the comedian Russ Abbott.

The Scotsman was wearing a massive kilt and a black beret adorned with long feathers. He was like something out of a book – I found it hard to believe that this was his everyday attire. He took us to the stables to see the three horses we had bought, who all looked well.

Then the Scotsman suddenly hissed, 'Keep still, everyone!' We froze, and right in front of us there suddenly materialised a big and beautiful brown Scottish stag with huge horns. It was a fantastic beast to see, but we were warned that it could be aggressive, and we stood in awe, very still, as the animal slowly stalked off past us away towards the mountains.

We were free now to load the horses on board the box trailer and set off on our way back to England. Uncle Matt was a lot happier now, which was a relief. But then my ears became uncomfortable, and started to pop. The road narrowed, until it was only six feet wide. The second driver got out the map and studied it. 'We are going the wrong way,' he announced. 'We are heading towards Glasgow.'

Uncle Matt stopped the Landrover. Nobody said a word. The three of us sat in complete silence. But then the other driver said, 'Look to your left, Antony. It's a beautiful lake'.

Uncle Matt spoke then, and his voice sounded a bit odd. 'Don't look to your right, Antony. It must be a thousand foot drop down there'. And it was only then that we realised that the road we'd been driving up, with beautiful views of snowy mountains in the distance, was on a mountain, and had landed us in a spot that looked simultaneously like heaven and hell.

We had ended up perched atop a huge dam, with a sheer drop below. At that point a shepherd appeared, herding more than 500 sheep, which were all trying to push past us along the road. The sheep were jumping on the top of the Land Rover and box trailer, and pushing against the concrete walls on either side of the dam. It was mayhem.

Uncle Matt asked the shepherd for help. 'Could you direct us to the English border, please?'

'You English people,' the shepherd announced disparagingly, 'Need to find out a bit more about Scotland before you head up here'. He told us that if we kept going we would soon find the next road back to Ayr – which we did, but only after another two hours.

Eventually we found the main road, and a sign directing us to the English border. Uncle Matt stopped the Land Rover for petrol. We went into a cafe nearby. 'I'm so hungry,' I announced, 'That I could eat a horse'.

'Well, we've got three in the trailer,' laughed the second

driver.

We ate fish and chips instead, and then fed and watered our new horses. We passed through Checkpoint Charlie again, after some more thorough questioning from the military police. We were happy to be back on English soil.

At three in the afternoon, near Carlisle, we stopped at a village shop. All three of us were tired out, fed up, and feeling travel sick into the bargain. Uncle Matt bought some peppermints, and I went into a red phone box to call my Mum. 'Are you having a good time, Antony?' she asked.

'Scotland is a beautiful country,' I told her, 'But this trip is a total disaster. I never want to see another horse or pony as long as I live'.

Uncle Matt decided to head for the west side of Leeds, and on towards home. We still had many hours of driving in front of us though, and on impulse Matt went back into the shop and bought a whole box of Smiths crisps, along with six big bottles of Tizer and ten packets of all sorts of biscuits to keep us going.

'It's time to get moving now,' said Uncle Matt. But he was too tired to move, so the other driver took over, and off we went. Surely it could only be a smooth ride home now, after all we had been through?

We got back on the motorway, heading towards Manchester. We stopped there at a service station, but suddenly the horses started whinnying and kicking inside the box. The creatures were desperate for exercise and had terrible cramps in their legs.

We'd parked by all the big trucks, and we all worked together to get the horses out of the box trailer and give them hay and water and walk them around as quickly as we could. And then we hit another problem – we moved two of the horses back into the trailer but the third simply refused to go in.

Luckily, a truck driver came to our aid. He put his huge meaty arms and hands around the horse's rear end and with one shove the animal was back in his box, as we all watched in amazement.

The truckie then noticed that the Land Rover was leaking oil, so he checked the engine and repaired the leak. Uncle Matt thanked him, and offered to pay him for his help. 'Tell you what,' he replied, 'You can buy me a burger and meet the other truckers'.

We went into the cafe to find that the truckers were watching TV. 'We can't go now,' said Uncle Matt, 'Coronation Street is on'. So we spent a pleasant hour with the truckers, eating egg and chips washed down with plenty of cups of tea.

By the time we left, all three of us were feeling a lot better. 'We're off to see the Wizard,' we began to sing as we set off again, 'The wonderful Wizard of Oz'.

But soon time soon began to drag. We were finding it hard to stay awake and Uncle Matt wanted to stop for the night. But the other driver told Matt that he would drive the last one hundred and fifty miles instead, that Matt and I could sleep, and he'd wake us when we got close to home. So finally, we made it back. I fell asleep in Mum's arms, and slept at Ashtree House for the night.

I didn't wake up until eleven o'clock the next morning. 'Hello, young man,' said my Dad. 'Mum has got your favourite breakfast ready'.

On the table stood a steaming bowl of Scott's porridge oats. 'Oh no,' I groaned, 'You can give it to the horses.' I had had more than enough of Scotland after all our adventures (although it is of course a wonderful place, in case any Scots are reading this!)

On that very morning my new surgical shoes had finally arrived in the post. The two day trip to Scotland had marked the end of my lonely ordeal, and I was at last able to go back to school.

I can still remember my first World Cup – it was the start of my love affair with football. I was still only seven years old, and I was very excited that Nanny and Grandad Evans had invited Mum, Dad, Julie and I to watch the big match at their home in Tuckton, Bournemouth.

Nanny and Grandad created a special World Cup tea party in their dining room, and we all sat together glued to their small television screen.

The match started. The atmosphere was tense. England were playing Germany - the Germans scored first and there was a lot of shouting in response, 'They were off side!' 'The Ref must be blind!' 'Boo!'

Nanny came at that point in and asked, 'Anybody for more tea and cake?' Nobody answered her, poor lady. We all just sat staring at the TV, waiting for England to score. It was a long game, and although I was excited I was also really tired, so my Mum scooped me up and sat me on her knee.

It is hard to describe the tension in that room – the echo of the 98,000 fans (including the Queen herself!) at Wembley Stadium. When the England goal we all hoped for happened at last, Mum jumped in the air for joy, and I flew off her lap and landed on the table, with jam from the cakes splattered all over my face.

Nanny took me into the kitchen to clean me up and back in the lounge, to everyone's pride and joy, England scored again. Everybody was celebrating as England won the World Cup for the first time ever with a score of 4-2. Football was my new passion, and I was hooked.

In September of 1966, not long before my eighth birthday, we moved to another house. It had belonged to my Grandad Cook – he had originally bought it to accommodate the riding instructor from his riding school, but he sold it on to us.

It was a newish house, facing towards the fields where Grandad kept his horses. The garden was overgrown, and Mum soon had plans to sort it out. I liked the house, and made new friends in the area very quickly. We still live in the same house today!

One evening my sister Julie and I went to the fairground at Ringwood Carnival with our Uncle Matt and some of his friends. Julie was allowed to go off with her friend, and I stayed with Uncle Matt. To Matt's surprise (and mine) I proved to be a natural with the air rifle - I scored very highly from the start. The lady behind the counter was getting a little red in the face.

'You are winning all the prizes,' she said. How on earth does a little boy like you know how to shoot an air rifle so well?'

'He's a natural,' said Uncle Matt cheerfully. Then he turned to me, grinning, 'Your Mum and Dad are going to throttle me. You have won yourself eight goldfish!'

I stared transfixed at my prizes. Each fish was swimming in a clear plastic bag full of water with a string handle attached to it. Suddenly Julie arrived back at our sides with her friend in tow. 'Look what I have won!' she yelled. 'Four goldfish!'

Poor Uncle Matt had to find a way to get twelve fish safely home. We got into the car. Julie held two bags, and I held two more. Two goldfish were tied onto the inside front mirror. Which still left us with six.

Uncle Matt's friend took two fish and tied them onto the side lights of his Bubble Car. Another of Matt's friends hung two on his Vespa Scooter handle bars. Then Matt hung the final pair of fish onto his own side mirrors. Luckily you could get away with a thing like that in those days – try it today and the police would stop you before you could say, 'Jack Robinson'!

We all started off on the journey back home, in a convoy with our twelve new goldfish. Mum and Dad had quite a surprise to see what we had brought back from the fair with us. 'Well,' said Mum, 'At least we can have fish for tea tomorrow'.

We had to put the fish into a bucket, because we had nowhere else for them to go. The next day Dad started building a pond in the back garden, and Mum worked on making borders for the flower beds. Just one week later the garden was transformed, with a pond full of goldfish surrounded by beautifully coloured flowers all complemented by a rich green lawn.

Chapter Four
A Family Holiday

Christmas was approaching, and Mum took Julie and I to see Father Christmas at Beales Department Store in Bournemouth. I sat on his lap and he asked me what I wanted.

'I would like a Dalek suit,' I told him.

He looked at me and smiled. 'Well, young man,' he said. 'I will talk to Dr Who myself about this one. I will try my very best for you. Merry Christmas!'

He'd better get me one, I thought to myself. I still need to get my own back on Julie for making me miss the end of the Dr Who film because of her stupid ballet lesson. That had happened a whole year ago, but I had not forgotten.

Christmas Day arrived, and Julie and I were breathless with excitement. We walked into the lounge very slowly, speechless to find nearly the whole of the floor covered with presents. When I saw so many gifts I hoped against hope that my dream had come true. I started to rip the Christmas wrapping paper off the first box and my eyes lit up with joy when I saw what I had uncovered. 'WOW!' I said. 'It's a red Dalek suit!'

The Dalek suit was made out of plastic. I put it on over my head and it nearly touched the ground. Then with my left hand I gripped the exterminator gun, and in my right hand I held a stick with a small plastic saucer on the end. It looked just like the plunger my Dad used when the sink was blocked.

It was perfect. I chased my sister all around the house in my new outfit, and exterminated her (although only in my imagination). I felt satisfied that she had finally been properly punished for taking up ballet dancing lessons.

Later that day Grandad and Nanny Cook arrived, to join us for Christmas dinner and Mum's special home-made Christmas pudding with cream and custard. After the meal everybody fell asleep in their armchairs, snoring their heads off with their Christmas cracker hats tipping down onto their noses. Eventually they woke up and we all put on our coats and made our way to Ashtree House for a Christmas tea. The whole family - cousins, aunties and uncles – always joined in the Ashtree House Christmas tea party because Grandad loved Christmas, and he relished the opportunity to get all the family together.

There was much fun and games during the afternoon. We watched films and played music, talked and laughed and danced. I loved Christmas.

In the summer holidays of 1967, Mum and Dad took Julie and I on holiday to Brixham in Devon. We started off at 6am.

'Now, you two,' Mum said. 'We're going to have a competition to see how many signposts you can spot on the way'.

'Signpost!' I shouted. That was one to me.

But then Julie started shouting her head off. 'Signpost! Signpost! Signpost!'

I hit her with my Beano comic. 'Mum!' I wailed. 'Julie is cheating! It's so unfair! She's covering my eyes with her hands so I can't see the signposts!'

Mum started to get annoyed with us. 'Listen,' she said crossly. 'Any more nonsense and you will both get into big trouble'.

Mum separated us, Julie on the left and me on the right side of the back seat. Nature was calling now, and I let go with a big bang of wind in the car. It was a bad one. Dad stopped the car, and Mum and Julie opened the windows wide.

'Antony,' said Mum, 'How could you? And you can take that grin off your face right now, you naughty little boy. Or else'.

Eventually we arrived at our destination. Brixham was a fantastic fishing village, with a harbour and a long stretch of walkway to the lighthouse. It was all very scenic – we could already spy the fishermen on their trawlers mending their nets, seagulls hovering over them screeching and squawking, hoping for a taste of fish.

We continued the long drive up a steep hill to the Devon Courts holiday flats, our home for the week. We hurried into our flat and straight out onto the balcony which had a fantastic panoramic view of the walkway to the Brixham lighthouse.

The next day Mum and Dad had arranged a visit to the famous village of Cockington. This was another lovely setting – small cottages with tea gardens, tourists enjoying rides on horses and traps. I was walking along ahead of my parents and spotted a sign fixed to a garden wall. It was beautifully hand-painted onto a wooden log plaque, although I could not understand what it said because the writing was in Old English.

Innocently I took a photo of the sign. Dad came over and asked if I was having a good time. 'Dad,' I said. 'I have just taken a photo of that sign. It's lovely. But what does it say?'

Dad went very red in the face and began to laugh. 'What's he done now?' asked Julie condescendingly.

Then Mum came over. 'What are you laughing about?' she enquired. 'What did you take a picture of, Antony?'

'That nice sign,' I said. 'It is lovely writing, Mum. But I couldn't read it. What does it say?'

Mum tried to keep a straight face. She whispered into my ear. 'It says TOILETS'.

I felt so embarrassed that I started to cry. Soon I was bawling my head off in front of all the onlookers, which soon stopped my family from giggling at me. Once I calmed down we all went to a teashop, where we shared a pot of tea and some Devon scones with jam and thick lumpy clotted cream. The wasps buzzed around us, trying to eat the jam before we did.

The next day Mum and Dad took Julie and I for another outing, to the Babbacombe model village in Torquay. It was amazing – four acres of delightful gardens, models and displays, with hundreds of animated models, vehicles and people, and miniature railways.

I spotted a little house no bigger than my hands. It had a

tiny working television set showing programmes in black and white. It was all rather wonderful. We spent nearly half a day there. I loved the idea of seeing everything in miniature, thinking how it would suit me if the whole world was scaled down like this.

The next day we went fishing. At the tackle shop, Dad bought Julie and I a fishing rod each with bubble floats attached, and we found ourselves a great spot to fish from the rocks overlooking Brixham harbour.

Julie and I started a fishing competition. Whoever caught the most fish would win a bag of sweets. Julie kept catching small fish and throwing them back in the water. 'It's not fair,' I complained. 'Julie keeps catching the same old fish over and over'.

Mum called us to say that tea was served. She laid a table cloth over the grassy bank. There were fish paste sandwiches with slices of cucumber, jam butties and a whole packet of Royal Scots round biscuits – and of course a flask of tea, to wash it all down.

I wanted a Wagon Wheel for pudding, but they had melted so badly that Mum suggested I used one for bait instead. I did so, and to my pride I caught a whopper – a two pound dogfish. Mum gave Julie the prize though, because she had caught more, even though all her fish together would not have weighed anything near as much as my big one.

The day was almost over now. We walked around a few shops, and then found a little pub where we could eat our evening meal. Dad found a table in the beer garden. It was very cosy, with tables fashioned out of beer barrels with umbrellas fixed to them. We tucked into our food, watching the Morris Dancers prancing around us in an impromptu show. They looked funny, hitting their wooden pole sticks together, dressed in white with small white bells sewn onto their outfits. As the dancers finished and we got up to head back to the flat, I felt a sharp pain shoot through my right leg – the short, bad leg – from my knee to my ankle.

I managed to stand up, but I could not walk. I was crying out in agony. Mum and Dad helped me back to the flat, and Mum said that I shouldn't worry, as it was probably just growing pains. It was getting late now. Mum gave me an Aspro tablet to ease the pain before I went to bed. It worked and I got to sleep, but I woke again shortly after midnight. I had more discomfort than I had ever experienced before – my right leg felt as though someone was twisting and stretching it viciously.

Mum ran a hot bath, and Dad lifted me into it to soak my legs in the warmth. It was three am by now, but finally the pain eased. I went back to bed and slept like a log. It was nine in the morning before I woke and called for a cup of tea.

Julie brought the tea. 'How are you now, little brother?' she asked. 'You were in a bad way last night'.

'I'll be fine' I told her. And I really thought I would be.

However, I soon started to feel unwell again. We had a roast lunch, but afterwards I had stabbing pains all over my hip and knee joints, and I could not walk without bending almost double. My hands and fingers were swelling, and even my neck was hurting. Mum was distressed from seeing me in so much pain, and she began to cry. We made our way back to the holiday flat, where all she could do was give me another Aspro tablet to ease the pain.

I think my parents must have felt as bad as I did at that point. So far our lives had been relatively unaffected by my disability. I knew that I had Morquio's Syndrome. I'd had that awful moment of realisation at Great Ormond Street some years before, seeing the other disabled children and realising that I was one of them. We shared the same destiny.

But I was lucky enough to be part of a secure loving family, and my life so far had not been too hard. To a large degree I was just an ordinary little boy, who enjoyed school and who had fun with his friends. There had been minor inconveniences, such as the problems with my surgical shoes, and of course I had never liked being so small for my age. I knew that being disabled was not going to be easy, but so far life had treated me well.

This sudden onslaught of pain, then, was a harsh reminder of reality. Coming out of the blue, in the middle of our family holiday, it was a wake-up call for us all, an indication that my disability was going to have more impact on my life – and on all of our lives – than we had previously realised. And worse was to follow....

For now, though, Mum sprang into action, ringing Dr Cantlie to explain what had happened. He told Mum that they should bring me straight home, 'I think Antony has developed a serious problem related to his disability,' the doctor warned.

Mum rang Grandad then, to say that I had been taken seriously ill and that we would be back late that same evening. During the journey back from Brixham I felt as if my whole body was burning, although at the same time both of my legs felt completely numb.

I was in the back of the car, crying out in pain, and Mum sat beside me, cradling me in her arms. After about an hour I dropped off, and slept fitfully through the journey. At 11pm we finally reached home, and Mum took me straight upstairs to bed.

Dr Cantlie arrived soon after. He gave me a thorough check, looking over my legs, hands, ribs, feet and neck. He also took a blood sample and gave me a pain-killing injection.

'It's not looking good,' he told my Mum. 'I'll make you an appointment to see Mr Lloyd Roberts at Great Ormond Street as soon as possible'.

'How long do you think it will take to come through?' asked my Mum.

'About a week,' replied Dr Cantlie. 'Antony can go back to school in the meantime, if he feels able'.

It was the start of the new term, and I did go back to school, although I was very tired and did not feel at all well. I was finding it very hard to keep up with my school work. I couldn't concentrate, or even grip a pen or pencil to draw or write. Every bone in my body felt as though it was cracking. I felt like giving up, and at my lowest point I hoped that I would just rot in bed until I died. I was a very miserable boy indeed.

In the middle of September a letter arrived from Great Ormond Street, with an appointment to see Mr Lloyd

Roberts on October 12th, just a few days before my ninth birthday.

I carried on going to school each day, and began to catch up with my reading, although I still had problems gripping a pen or pencil. I was looking forward to my birthday now – Mum had promised that I could have a party, and invite my school friends to celebrate with us. But first I had to see the specialist.

One day, the Junior School headteacher, Mr Hackett, asked my parents and I to come and see him. It was late afternoon, after school had finished for the day, when we assembled in his office.

'If Antony has to stay in hospital,' said Mr Hackett, 'I will make sure he has a home tutor to keep up with his school work until he is well again'.

Mum and Dad were lost for words. I was speechless too – it had not occurred to me until this point that I might have to stay in hospital. Mum looked over at me. 'Don't worry, Antony,' she said. 'Just hold on, and be a very brave little boy until we hear what the specialist has to say'.

Chapter Five
Great Ormond Street Hospital

The 12th of October soon arrived. The journey seemed just the same as the first time two years earlier; the long trek to London by train and then to the hospital by taxi, and the thick smog hanging in the air when we arrived.

When we got to Great Ormond Street we made our way to the same waiting room as before. I was very quiet, biting my fingernails with nerves. Finally the nurse called me into the consulting room, and asked me to undress and put on a white gown ready to be examined. I sat on a tall bed and waited, feeling sick with anticipation and nerves.

When Mr Lloyd Roberts finally arrived, he was surrounded by a group of young student doctors and his secretary. 'Hello, Antony,' he greeted me, as if it had only been five minutes since we last met. 'I hear you have not been very well. Bad pains in your legs since your holiday in Devon, eh?'

He smiled as he started to examine me, moving my arms and legs, and all the time talking to the students at his side, showing them my X-rays in a light box screen.

His secretary was keeping up with his speech, taking notes of what he said. The consultant noted the big bone sticking out of my right knee. He said I had an overgrown femur. He turned and spoke to my parents, who had been waiting and listening anxiously.

'Antony will need an operation on this overgrown femur,' he told them. 'All the pains he has been experiencing recently are growing pains. But unfortunately, due to his condition, the bones are growing wrongly, which is why the pain is so severe'.

Mr Lloyd Roberts decreed that I should be admitted to hospital as soon as possible, to undergo the operation. Provided they could find a bed for me, the operation would be scheduled for before Christmas, he said.

A nurse was then summoned, to show Mum, Dad and I around the ward where I would be staying. I found it a really upsetting experience, as the beds were filled with children suffering from different disabling conditions, all of them extremely severe.

I met several doctors and nurses, who all seemed to come from foreign countries. They were all very kind, but I found it hard to understand what some of them were saying. Then a tiny girl approached me. 'Hello, my name is Bev,' she said. 'Would you like to play a game of tiddly winks with me, Antony?' I was petrified, speechless with fear, because the girl was very badly disabled. I couldn't answer her because I was so scared of how she looked, and I was unable to explain why because I did not want to be rude.

Great Ormond Street Hospital was a huge building, many storeys high. The ward that I would be staying on was on the top floor, with a view over the skyscrapers in the heart of London. We met the Sister in charge of the ward, who was lovely. She showed me where my bed would be and promised Mum and Dad that they would all take good care of me when I came to hospital.

It was soon time to leave. We were due to catch the four o'clock train from Waterloo, and arrived at the station a little early. We sat down on a bench on the station platform. Nearby was a man selling bird seed for people to feed the pigeons. Mum bought me some seeds and I sat and watched as one greedy pigeon gobbled up everything I fed him.

Suddenly a road sweeping machine came along the platform, driven by a railwayman. As he passed us sweeping up the rubbish, he swept up my pigeon too. I could hear the pigeon being crushed to pieces inside the huge machine.

'Hey Mister,' I shouted to the man angrily. 'You owe me a shilling for all the bird seed I just fed to that pigeon!' The railwayman just kept on driving.

As we waited at the station I noticed that a lot of the women walking around looked like clones, with short dyed hair parted to the left, and heavy eye make up with long dark false lashes. I realised that they were all imitating Twiggy, the incredible supermodel. London was a new and glamorous world, and everyone there seemed to want to keep up to date with the new styles. Back in Christchurch, I'm not sure anyone would have known what the new styles were, or would have cared if they did.

We were all tired and relieved when we arrived home. I was still feeling unwell, but I forced myself to go back to school the next morning. I had decided to work even harder than usual, because I knew that soon I would be in hospital, and I didn't want to fall too far behind with my school work.

My birthday dawned. I had a party at home, and invited some school friends. We had the usual party fare – sausage rolls, pork pies, sandwiches and scotch eggs, followed by jelly and ice-cream, all varieties of biscuits and a special birthday cake, made by my Mum. It was emblazoned with my nickname, Noddy, and it had nine candles shining on the top.

I was in pain during the party: my right leg was playing me up again, but I put a brave face on things, and all my friends were very kind. When the party was over and only my family were around, I sat down heavily. My rib cage and legs were hurting badly.

Julie helped me up to my room, where I lay on the bed staring at the ceiling, unable to think about anything except hospital. I was very scared about the operation. One day, the dreaded letter letter arrived. I felt sick with nerves as Mum spoke, 'Mr Lloyd Roberts has booked you in for an operation on Thursday 14th December 1967'.

'I will be away for Christmas!' I cried out. Mum did her best to reassure me; 'Whatever happens,' she said, 'You will be in less pain after the operation. And soon you will be back home again'.

The letter made me late for school, and as soon as I arrived the music teacher, Mrs Tickner, asked if she could have a word with me. She wanted me to play tambourine in the school Christmas play, 'Toad of Toad Hall'. I knew that she saw this as an honour, and in fact it did me a lot of good, because all the rehearsals took my mind off the forthcoming operation.

On the designated evening, near the end of term, all our parents arrived to see the show. I really enjoyed playing the tambourine for the special sound effects and for the first time in ages I did not feel any pain. Looking back,

I think this must have been because I was so focused on the performance, concentrating on making sure that everyone enjoyed the show.

The concert went brilliantly. At the end there was loud applause and catcalls of, 'More, more!' The Headteacher, Mr Hackett, took the stage. 'What a fantastic show our children have put on for us,' he said. 'I would like to thank each and every one of you for all your support'.

'And also,' he continued, 'One of our pupils, Antony Evans, is leaving us for a short while to stay at Great Ormond Street. He is due to have an operation on his leg. I would like to give him best wishes on behalf of our school, and to tell him that we all hope he gets well and comes back to us very soon'.

Everybody started to clap again, even louder than before. I could feel myself going red in the face, I was so embarrassed to be the centre of attention.

On the Monday, my last day at school, I had another embarrassing surprise. One of my classmates, the girl who always sat next to me, leapt on me and gave me a whopping kiss on the lips. I had never experienced anything like this before, and all I could think about was how she could not have cleaned her teeth that morning. Her breath nearly knocked me out.

She was very sweet, though. 'Antony,' she said, 'You are my very best friend. I will keep your seat warm until you get well again'. My friends started to shout and call out, 'Antony's got a girlfriend. Antony's got a girlfriend!'

I ignored them all, put my head down and got on with my work. Soon enough it was the end of the day, and time to say goodbye to all my friends and teachers. Somehow I got through it without breaking down in tears, but it was a close call.

The next day I was admitted to Great Ormond Street Hospital. I was scheduled to have a supracondylar osteotomy to my right leg that was badly bent and twisted. The operation was due to take place on the morning of Thursday 14th December.

An hour before the operation was due to take place I lay in my bed, staring out of the window. I was scared and very homesick but I knew I had no choice but to go ahead with the operation, and that I had to be brave for the sake of my Mum and Dad.

I was wheeled down to the next floor on a trolley, and Mr Lloyd Roberts came to talk to me. 'Now, young Antony,' he said, 'We are going to give you something to make you go to sleep. When you wake up you will be back in your ward'.

He was right. I woke up in the middle of the night, back in the ward. Apparently, the operation had taken seven hours, although I had no notion of time passing. The ward was confusing – babies were crying in their ventilators, watched over by night nurses. I managed to lift myself up to sitting. I could see my right leg completely encased in plaster, and my left leg in a half plaster. Inconveniently, Mother Nature was calling.

'Nurse,' I called out.

A nurse came over. 'Hello, Antony. I see you have

woken up at last. What can I help you with?'

'I need a wee,' I told her.

'I'll get you a glass bottle,' said the nurse. She soon brought the bottle, and I relieved myself, but I was concerned when I saw that my urine was very brown.

'Don't worry,' said the nurse. 'That is the effects of the anaesthetic.'

Another nurse arrived, who checked my pulse, temperature and blood pressure. Everything was normal, they said. Later the night sister arrived, and she told me that although I was pain free now it would soon start to hurt again, because the surgeon had taken away a large piece of bone from my femur.

'It will take a month to heal,' she said. 'You won't be fully mobile again for a while. But we do have pain relief to help you while you are getting better'.

The next day I was woken up by the nurses at 6am and told that I was going to have a bed bath. I was half naked as they pushed me over onto my side. 'Wow,' said a nurse. 'You have got huge bedsores on your bottom. We will have to put some baby oil on – that will sort them out'.

They oiled my bum, and then smothered me in baby powder to keep the sores from returning. I stunk as if I had just come back from a doggy parlour. But then I was distracted by the pain, which had returned with a vengeance, just as the night sister had warned.

I was given strong painkillers, and soon it was breakfast

time. The food arrived on a trolley, and there was all sorts to choose from – cereal, toast, bacon or eggs, and tea or milk to drink. Afterwards I had to get dressed. But the plaster on my legs would not accommodate my trousers, so the nurses had to find some large trousers, then cut the legs off them to fit me. They did a good job.

Later the same day Mr Lloyd Roberts came to see me again. 'How are you today, Antony?' he asked.

'I am in a lot of pain,' I told him. 'And I am wondering why my left leg is in half plaster with all these bandages'.

'Your left leg was straining and slightly bending,' the doctor told me. 'We just had to manipulate it. But the right leg, the short one, had a big bone sticking out of the femur, and we had to remove that'.

'Will I have to stay in hospital for Christmas?' I asked.

'We"ll see how you get on,' said Mr Lloyd Roberts. 'I'll make a decision when I see you next, on Tuesday 19th December'.

Late that afternoon, a nurse approached me. 'I've got good news for you,' she said. 'Mr Lloyd Roberts has asked me to move you into a private room with just one other boy. It will help you recover more quickly – you can rest without being distracted by all the other children and babies on the ward'.

Just then my Mum and Dad arrived. I hugged them both tightly, and cried with joy. We had only been apart a short time, but I had missed them so much.

Once I had calmed down, I turned to my Mum and asked her, 'Where does the sun set, Mum?'

'Why do you want to know that, Antony?' she asked.

'So I know where you all are when I go to sleep,' I told her.

Both my parents stared at me for a moment. Then Dad said, 'The bed in your new private room faces north. If you look out through the window on your left, that is the South West, where we live and where the sun sets'.

The visit from my Mum and Dad soon ended, but after that I didn't feel so alone again. When it was time for bed each evening, I looked out of the window as Dad had instructed and in my heart I said a silent 'Goodnight,' to every member of my family. Each morning when I awoke I silently greeted them too. Knowing where they were, and that they were thinking of me as I was of them, helped to give me courage and hope throughout those dark and difficult days in the hospital.

It was almost Christmas time and my Dad went home on the train, but Mum stayed on in London because Christmas was so close. She found a place in a small Bed and Breakfast nearby. Before she left that evening she asked if there was anything I would like her to buy me from the shops.

'Yes please, Mum,' I said. 'I would like a small silver Christmas tree to go on my bedside locker'.

Mum took her mission very seriously, and started her

search in London the next morning. I sat in my bed, listening to the radio. Soon a little boy in a wheelchair came to see me. 'Hello,' he said. 'I have got polio. What have you got?'

'I'm Antony,' I told him. 'I have got Morquio's syndrome. And what is your name?'

'William,' he replied. 'Sorry, I have got to go now'.

With that, William wheeled himself back to his ward, and I never saw him again.

Every hour for the rest of that day, nurses checked my pulse and took my temperature and blood pressure. After one of these visits, a nurse left a chart on the end of my bed, showing the rise and fall of my pulse rate and temperature over the hours. I decided to have a good look before she came back to fetch it. I had just managed to get to the end of the bed and was perusing the chart, written on tenth of an inch graph paper, covered with lines and dots going up and down, when suddenly, I jumped to hear a voice behind me, 'Nosey!'

I turned around to see the Night Sister. 'Shut your eyes,' she said. 'I have a surprise for you'.

When I opened my eyes a moment later I saw my Mum standing next to my bedside locker, on which was perched the small silver Christmas tree I had wished for. It was beautiful, decorated with tiny red and blue balls. I could hardly believe my eyes.

Mum told me that she'd had great difficulty trying to find a small silver Christmas tree in central London. It meant a lot to me that my mother had worked so hard to track down that tree for me, and I still have it now, forty-five years on. Every Christmas the little silver tree comes out on display, and it reminds me of all the children at Great Ormond Street Hospital, and the doctors and nurses who work there.

On the 19th December, Mr Lloyd Roberts came to see me as he had promised. 'Well, Antony,' he said. 'You have been through a lot, and you are a very brave little boy. I would like you to stay in hospital for a little while longer. Hopefully you can go home for a few days over Christmas, but I am not sure about that yet; we will have to wait and see'.

Every night after that I addressed the little Christmas tree that stood on my locker. 'Please,' I begged. 'Please, please let me go home for Christmas'.

My wish came true – I was allowed home on December 23rd. My Mum and Dad came to collect me, with my Auntie Joyce and Uncle David (who were not actually relatives but close friends of the family – Uncle David worked with my Dad in the Fire Service). It was late when we got back, but it felt so good to be back in my own bed.

The next morning, however, I woke up in terrible discomfort. I called out for the nurse before I realised that today was Christmas Eve, and I was in my own home. The pain was in my right leg again, and I was soon crying out in agony. Mum gave me painkillers, but they had no effect, and so my parents called Dr Cantlie.

The doctor gave me an injection of morphine and said, 'This will only last four hours, I'm afraid, Antony. I'm very sorry that I can't do more for you'. He told my

Mum to phone Great Ormond Street and ask for advice.

When Mum spoke to the Ward Sister, she explained how I had awoken in severe pain and asked her for advice. The Sister told my mother that she should crush up some codeine tablets with a spoon to make a thin powder, and then mix that into a large glass of cold water. That would stop the pain, she said, but only for six hours.

As soon as I began to drink, I felt calmer and the agony began to recede. I just about got through the day, and in the evening Dad's friend Arthur came to visit me dressed up as Father Christmas. I enjoyed this, but at the same time longed for Boxing Day when I would get back to the comfort of the hospital. My leg was hurting again as the painkillers wore off, and I found it very hard to bear. I had been so excited about coming home for Christmas, but I hadn't bargained for all this.

The next morning was Christmas Day, and when I woke up Julie was sitting on my bed.

'What do you want?' I asked her.

My sister took my grumpiness to mean that I was still sleepy. 'Come on, Antony,' she said impatiently. 'I've been waiting for you. It's time to open our presents'.

'No,' I said.

'What do you mean?' she asked. 'Why not?'

'Just leave me alone!' I shouted at her. 'I have wet my bed. I haven't got a present for you, or for Mum and Dad. I blame myself, because I am disabled, and I have just had an operation, and I am in pain, and it hurts more than you could ever imagine. So just go away!'

I was alone then, as I had asked, but it didn't make me feel any better. I could hear Julie crying from where I lay. So I called Mum to help me get washed and dressed, and went downstairs to join my family. Nothing was said about my outburst.

I had lots of cards and presents. There was even a card from the girl who sat next to me in the classroom, the same one who had embarrassed me by kissing me on the last day that I had been at school. Usually I would have loved to open everything, but I was distracted by the pain, which nagged at me and seemed to drag all the pleasure out of my life.

I was not my usual self at all, and all I could think about was wanting to go back to the hospital as soon as I could. I knew that they would make me comfortable there.

It was time for breakfast, and Dad wheeled me into the kitchen. Mum had made her traditional Christmas fry-up, but suddenly I felt sick and before I knew it I had thrown up all over the floor. It was a horrible stinking mess, and it seemed to me that life had become a horrible stinking mess too. I lost control then, and began to shout and cry. I was swearing at my family, yelling that I wished I was dead, and that I had never been born. 'Why am I like this?' I kept bawling. I threw what was left of my breakfast across the table. 'Help me! Help me!' I shouted.

I really felt as though I come to the limit of my capability. I could not cope any more, but nevertheless the anger I felt was mingled with shame at my behaviour, because the last thing I really wanted was to upset my family.

Julie got up then, and came over to my side of the table. She hugged me tightly. 'Listen, Antony,' she said. 'You will get through this. It will take time, and it won't be easy, but you must not give up. You will be back to school again, and you will feel as right as rain'.

Mum and Dad were watching us, and I could see that they were both feeling very emotional. 'Your sister is right,' my Dad said. 'You will be okay'.

It helped a lot to know that my family loved me so much, no matter what I did or said. They understood my predicament. I made an effort to calm down and put a brave face on things, and later on Grandad and Nanny Cook came over for Christmas dinner. Mum and Dad had cooked the meal together, and they looked worn out from the stress of the morning as we all sat down at the table to eat.

Grandad had a surprise in store. 'When you come for our Christmas tea at Ashtree House this afternoon,' he said. 'We are going to play Bingo. And Antony can call out the numbers'.

I smiled at Grandad. I was pretty excited about the prospect of being a Bingo caller. I was still not feeling well, but I managed to eat part of my Christmas dinner, and some Christmas pudding. I was too weak to pull my Christmas cracker properly though, and had to use two hands to do it. A mighty bang ensued, and out of the debris of the cracker fell a hat, a miniature pack of playing cards, and a piece of paper with a joke written on it.

'What kind of motorbike does Santa ride?' I read out. 'A Holly Davidson!'

'The jokes are getting worse each year,' said my Dad. 'Can't you think of a better joke than that?'

'Which football team does baby Jesus support?' I asked. 'Manger-ster United!' Everybody laughed at that one.

Christmas Day seemed to be settling into its normal pattern, after the upset of the morning. We went over to Ashtree House later in the afternoon, and played Bingo with all the cousins, aunties and uncles. I eventually fell asleep on the bingo board, while still calling out the numbers, and when I woke up I found myself on my bed at home. Finally, Boxing Day had arrived.

I was due to travel to London by train, and a carriage had been reserved for me and my wheelchair. An ambulance arrived at our door, to transport me to Christchurch train station, and several neighbours appeared to wave me off. I had very little energy at that point, but managed a weak smile in response.

We travelled by express train, in a first class carriage. The journey was much quicker this time, and when we arrived at Waterloo station another ambulance was waiting to transport me to Great Ormond Street. Eventually we reached the hospital, and I was safely installed back in my private room. The whole ward was covered in Christmas decorations, and all the children were happily sitting up in their beds, surrounded by their families. Everybody seemed to be having a jolly good time, including the nursing staff, who were as brilliant as usual, and even kinder and friendlier than they normally were, if such a thing was possible. I could tell from the scene around me (and from my own recent experiences) that it was not such a bad thing for children to spend Christmas in hospital, if that is where they need to be.

'Merry Christmas, Antony,' the ward sister said, by way of greeting. 'Would you like some Christmas cake?' But by this point I was so exhausted that I could not even reply, and I fell fast asleep.

While I was still asleep, my Mum and Dad had a meeting with the doctor and sister in the Ward Office. When I woke again I saw a nurse sitting on a chair by my bed. I thought it was my sister Julie at first, panicked when I saw that it was not, and started to call out for my Mum and Dad.

'Hello, Antony,' said the nurse. 'Don't worry. Your Mum and Dad are just talking to the doctor'.

'I feel as though my brain is playing tricks on me,' I told her. 'One minute I am at home, the next I am back here'. The nurse was sympathetic and I soon got a grip on myself.

When Mum and Dad reappeared, they told me that I would be staying in hospital for another twelve days to convalesce. After that I would need to learn to walk again. 'The good news is,' Mum said, 'You're nearly on the mend'.

'The bad news,' I retaliated, 'Is that I'm driving everyone around the bend!'

Dad went home by train that day, and Mum stayed on again. This time though, she stayed with a friend. The next morning she brought me an Airfix model kit and some glue to build a B.O.A.C passenger plane. She also made me a twelve day calendar, so I could colour in the days I was staying.

Chapter Six
Convalescence

It was now the New Year of 1968. Two days later, I had to go back to the operating theatre, where I was given a general anaesthetic to have the stitches taken out of my leg and the plaster changed.

The next day, Dad came to visit. Mum was still staying with me in London, and when Dad visited Julie would go to Ashtree House to stay with Nanny and Grandad Cook until one of our parents came home. It was all planned with the precision of a military operation.

Dad was really pleased to see me looking better. I was moving all around the ward in my wheelchair, nearly knocking the nurses over as I careered in and out of my room. After a couple of hours had passed, Dad announced that he was off home. 'You're doing well, son,' he said. 'Only five days now before you're home. Cheerio for now'.

Before Dad left he gave Mum a train ticket to travel back to Christchurch the next day, because Julie was dancing in a big charity show at the Bournemouth Pavilion. The next morning Mum came into my room at half past ten, and I put on a brave face when she hugged me and left the hospital to embark on the long journey back home.

It must have been hard for my parents – Dad working two jobs and still making it up to London to visit me when he could, Mum dividing her time and attention between Julie and I. I didn't make a fuss because I knew Mum was doing her best for both of us. Mum told me later that she arrived home and caught a taxi to

Bournemouth Pavilion just before the curtain went up for the show, and that luckily she'd just managed to get a message to Julie to say that she was there.

The other problem that my family faced was the extra expense that was caused by my stay in hospital. We had a travel warrant through Hampshire County Council and initially this meant that we could apply for travel costs to and from Great Ormond Street to be reimbursed before or after the event. The rules changed however, and we were only allowed to apply for travel costs in advance – this was difficult for my parents to do as they often could not predict the dates of their journeys. In the end they just gave up claiming from the Council and shouldered all the expenses themselves.

One day, I had a surprise outing. The day sister popped her head around the door of my room and announced, 'You are going to Tadworth Court for the day, Antony. Don't worry, a nurse will be going with you'.

'Why are you sending me there?' I asked.

'It is the Great Ormond Street Hospital's Country Branch,' the sister replied. 'It's in Surrey, near Epsom Race Course. That's where they will teach you to walk again. Today you'll have some X-rays and be given a good look around'.

Obediently I lifted myself into my wheelchair and set off, pushed by the nurse who had been assigned to look after me. We made our way through the basement of the hospital into the car park, where a Variety Club Sunshine Bus was waiting to take me to Tadworth Court. It was still very early in the morning, because we were leaving in time to beat the London rush hour.

It was an hour before we got out of London, and were driving through Surrey. It was a warm day for early January, and the sun shone brightly. When we arrived at Tadworth Court we had to drive through the gatehouse entrance, and then the bus trundled up a short path to the beautiful house.

Tadworth Court is a Grade One listed mansion and a hidden secret, just yards from the main route into London. It was purchased by Great Ormond Street Hospital in 1926, and served as its country branch until 1983. It is a stunning building. That day was the first time I had seen the place, and the nurse and I both stood in the courtyard for a moment, gazing up at the mansion in front of us. There were stables and various other small buildings next to the main house.

I turned to the nurse. 'Will I be staying in the big mansion house to learn to walk again?' I asked.

She laughed. 'I'll show you around in a minute Antony,' she told me. 'First we have to register you for the day'.

We went into the main house then, and through to the registration room. I could see inside the main lounge as we passed, where there was a massive fireplace and an enormous wooden staircase. I was still trying to figure out where the wards were. Next I was wheeled through to the underground basement, which I found quite frightening. We stopped at the X-ray room, where several nurses laid me onto a special bed. They all wore blue lead jackets to protect them from the radiation.

The camera was aimed at my legs and hips. A lady in a white coat said gently, 'Now, Antony, we are going to take the X-rays. I want you to stay very still for me. You will have to be patient because we have to take lots of pictures of your legs, arms, neck, ribs, back, bottom, feet, toes, shoulders, hips and hands'.

The X-rays took several hours. When they were finally finished I had to stay on the bed for another hour, waiting. If they had not developed properly, I was told, the whole process would have to be gone through again.

Finally, the white-clad lady returned. 'Hello again, Antony,' she said. 'The X-rays all showed up well. The nurse will take you to ZMA ward now, to have your lunch before you go back to London'.

I was wheeled out through the basement and into what I was told was the 'Tadworth Court Magic Garden', then through a very long arched pathway. The place resembled an upmarket holiday camp. 'What do you think, Antony?' asked the nurse. 'This is where you will be learning to walk again'.

I realised that my ward would not be in the mansion house at all, but in another purpose-made building nearby. I was taken to the playroom first, where I sat in my wheelchair for lunch with the other children. The playroom was bordered by two long wards – ZMA for the boys and ZMB for the girls.

The sister in charge of both wards showed me around ZMA, and took me to see my bed and locker. 'This is where you will be staying when you are with us,' she said. 'I'll take you to the physiotherapy room now, and you can see the apparatus you will be using when you learn to walk again'.

I was wheeled from ZMA ward along another arched pathway to the physio room. It was housed in a tiny square building with two glass-panelled doors. I was introduced to an orthopaedic physiotherapist then. She said, 'Hello,' she said. 'We are going to be helping you to walk using these long walk cradle bars. And we will be helping you to bend your knee again by practising walking up and down on these small wooden stairs'.

After that, I was taken around the grounds of Tadworth Court. The place was fantastic! I could hardly believe my eyes, and was really looking forward to staying here. I already felt grateful to whoever it was who had decided to create a country branch for the Great Ormond Street Hospital.

All too soon, it was time to leave. The nurse and I travelled back in the Variety Sunshine Club bus, arriving very late because we were caught in the rush hour. I was starving, and someone managed to rustle me up some food, after which I spoke to my Mum on the phone in the nurses' office, telling her all about my day. I handed the receiver back to the nurse, and could still hear Mum on the line as they spoke together, 'I have not heard my son so happy for a long time'.

'Antony is a great fighter,' the nurse answered. 'He has not asked for a pain killer for the last few days – he is pain free now, and he is mobilising well'.

The next day, Dr Lloyd Roberts came to see me with his usual entourage of medical students and secretary. He was very pleased that I was feeling stronger and was pain-free. 'Well, young Antony,' he said, 'You'll be glad to know that the femur has completely healed now and you will be discharged tomorrow'.

I was delighted. Before I could leave though, various matters had to be sorted out with the hospital. My parents and I saw the consultant together, and he told them that he was very sorry that he had not been able to lengthen my right leg as he had hoped.

'The leg is not strong enough,' he told them, 'And we do not want to risk causing any further complications as he grows older. What we have done, though, is to move a large piece of bone from his femur. He will be standing straighter and walking better from now on'.

'Thank you,' said my Dad. 'And what happens now?'

'Antony won't be able to return to school yet,' Mr Lloyd Roberts replied. 'You should hear from my secretary by February regarding your son's transfer to Tadworth Court, our country branch in Surrey, where he will learn to walk again. Although, of course, all that will depend on when we have an available bed'.

The Sister and other nurses came to my room then, where there was an emotional farewell. It was hard to say goodbye to all the people who had cared for me during my long stay in hospital. I was keen to go home, but I knew I would miss the hospital routine, and I felt sad leaving all the other children behind.

I still had the plaster on my right leg, so a flat splint was fixed onto my wheelchair to rest the plastered leg on. Mum had booked the three of us into a First Class carriage on an express train from Waterloo to Christchurch. We arrived home late in the afternoon, and I felt instantly more comfortable.

The next morning my Mum rang my school, and spoke to Mr Hackett, the headteacher. He was delighted to hear that I was back home, but he said that unfortunately although he had applied to get me home tuition he had been turned down.

Mum was disappointed, but used her initiative to sort out an alternative course of action. She saw an advert for home tuition in our local paper, placed by a University student. Mum interviewed the girl, liked her, and consequently employed her to help me with my school work each day.

Time passed slowly. After a week I had taught myself to clamber up and down the stairs with my plastered leg, and even to crawl on the floor along to the lounge and kitchen. However, I was not allowed to put weight on the leg, because there was a risk that I could break the plaster and cause further problems.

Many of my school friends visited, and they all signed my plaster. I was given so many sweets by them, and from all my Aunties and Uncles, that I could not possibly eat them all. So I decided to sell them instead, and to donate the money to the local Guide Dogs for the Blind Association.

A few days later, a postman knocked. 'I've got a parcel for your son from the BBC,' he told Mum. 'Could you sign for it, please? And that's not all I have for him. Just take a look in here'.

Mum peeped inside the postman's sack, and was overwhelmed by what she saw. There were stacks of cards from my friends, wishing me better. I turned my attention to the parcel, which was indeed from the BBC.

It was two Corgi cars, with a note inside to say that I should have received this gift during my stay at Great Ormond Street.

I found out later that the BBC gave (and still give) gifts to all the children who are staying at Great Ormond Street Hospital over Christmas. I had missed out on my gift because I had gone home on Christmas Day, but now here it was! The Sister from my ward had given my home address to the BBC so that they could forward the parcel to me. Much better late than never.

The latest letter from Mr Lloyd Roberts' secretary arrived as expected in the first week of February. It announced that I would be admitted to stay at the Great Ormond Street Country Branch at Tadworth in Surrey on the 12th February 1968. When we arrived, we were greeted by a nurse, who took my parents and I through the magic garden to ward ZMA where I would be staying. Mum and Dad were amazed at the sight of the children clambering up trees, seemingly unbothered by the plaster casts on their legs.

We got to my bed and soon the Sister arrived to speak to my parents. She explained that I would be staying at Tadworth Court for at least twelve days, and that I would learn to walk again with a special physiotherapy programme. Hopefully I would be fully mobile, and able to return to school, in one month's time.

The first day of my stay I was left to settle in and acclimatise to my surroundings. On the second day I was wheeled to a small room to have the plaster cast removed from my leg. The specialist who cut the plaster off used a special tool; metal-cutting scissors just like the ones my Dad used for his plumbing work.

After the plaster was cut off, there was mess everywhere. My leg was a mess too, very thin and extremely itchy. I could see a big scar on my femur where the operation had taken place. I tried to touch it but it felt extremely raw, and a cold shiver travelled down my spine at the sensation. (The scar feels sore to this day, and as I write I imagine it is telling me, 'Don't forget to put me in the book, Antony!')

On the third day of my stay I spent most of my time with the physiotherapist. The next day I stayed on the ward, where I rested on my bed, although I was told to keep practising bending my leg. I was not expecting any visitors, but there was a surprise arrival.

'Uncle Matt!' I cried out when I saw him. 'What are you doing here?'

'Well, Antony,' said my Uncle. 'I knew you would be in hospital for a while, so I have brought you a Lion Annual and a Tiger Annual to keep you amused'. I was over the moon with these presents, and with seeing my Uncle – and I still have the books to this day.

Eventually, Uncle Matt announced that he had to go. 'Bye!' he called. 'Keep your hands off those nurses!' I squirmed with embarrassment, but couldn't help laughing. One thing was sure – life was never dull with Matt around!

A week later, I was starting to feel more mobile. I could manage a few steps up and down the ward on my crutches, and started to make friends with some of the other children.

Every morning at 6am the night nurses would wake us all up, so that they could change the bedsheets. The bed covers were made of nylon, the nurses used to get quite bad shocks from the static electricity when they changed the sheets. We children could hear the bed covers crackling, and the nurses shouting, 'Ouch! Ouch!' and it always made us laugh. It was a good show to start the day with.

One morning it began to snow, and the snow kept falling until there was a thick blanket of it on the ground outside. Some of the children were taken outside in their wheelchairs, where they had snowball fights with the nurses. It was great fun watching them through the windows, but I was happy to stay in the warm.

I started talking to an Indian girl, who told me her name was Jay. I felt very sorry for her, because she was laid out on her bed and couldn't move at all. She was wired up to what looked like a very painful contraption.

'I had to have my leg lengthened,' Jay told me. 'It was badly twisted, because it had been growing wrong'.

Jay was very brave, and I realised that I was not the only one having to cope with being away from home. There were many other children in the same position, and I was lucky that my parents visited so often. I was homesick, but I knew that my ordeal would soon be over.

One afternoon, the Matron came to see me. She was a big woman – she looked just like Hattie Jacques from the film, 'Carry On, Matron'.

'Jolly good,' she said vaguely. Then she looked at her

notes, all the while mumbling to herself, although I could not hear what she was saying as she had a pencil lodged in her mouth. Finally she spoke, 'It seems from the notes,' she said, 'That you have now completed your physiotherapy programme. Mr Lloyd Roberts will see you later today, to carry out a final examination'.

Was I really going home? I walked on my crutches to the playroom, where I could see through the window that the snow had all melted away now. I sat there for hours, until a nurse came to tell me to go to sit on my bed, because the doctor had arrived to see me.

Mr Lloyd Roberts was waiting by my bed, secretary in tow as usual. 'It looks from the notes as though you have done very well, Antony,' he said as he turned to me. 'How does it feel to be walking again?'

'My right leg is much more mobile now,' I told him, 'Although it still feels sore. And my back does not bend over as much as it used to. I am very grateful for what you have done for me'.

The doctor started talking to his secretary then. 'Antony Evans can be discharged tomorrow,' he said, 'The 25th February. I will need to see him again in six months at Great Ormond Street Outpatients Department, for a check-up'.

Once he had gone, the Day Sister came in. She told me that she had already spoken to my Mum and Dad and that they would be picking me up the next day. It was 6pm, supper time, and so I made my way to the playroom where we all ate our meals. I sat next to Jay, who was wheeled in on her bed to eat with us, and I told her that I was due to go home the following day. To my dismay, she started to cry.

'Don't do that!' I said. 'You'll start me off, and between us we might flood the playroom'.

Jay started to giggle then, 'You should be a comedian, Antony,' she said. 'By the way,' she went on, 'How old are you?'

'Ten this year,' I said. 'How old are you, Jay?'

'The same,' my friend told me.

The next morning I went into the playroom for breakfast. I knew I should be happy, because today I was going home for good, but I felt bad about leaving Jay behind, lying on her bed with pins stuck in her leg. I was very young, but my feelings for Jay were stronger than friendship – I really liked her, and I was going to miss her.

Jay was quiet too when she was wheeled in on her bed to have her breakfast. She called me over. 'Would you stay with me for a little while before you start packing?' she asked.

'Of course I will,' I said.

'I won't have anyone to talk to now that you're leaving,' said Jay.

'You never know Jay, your family could turn up to see you right now,' I said, trying to cheer her up.

Suddenly Jay's face lit up, and I turned around to see a crowd of people in the doorway behind me – my friend's entire family had arrived to visit! I made my way slowly back to my ward, leaving them alone together.

While I was packing my things, a lady appeared by my bedside. 'I'm Hanna,' she said. 'Jay's mother. I just wanted to say thank you for looking after my daughter'.

Before I left I went to Jay's room to give her a big hug. She passed me a letter then, and whispered in my ear, 'One day, when I'm older, I'm going to marry you'.

I smiled. 'Goodbye, Jay,' I said.

It was time now. I was put into a wheelchair, and wheeled by a nurse through the long paths, under the archways, to the main part of Tadworth Court, where Mum and Dad were waiting to take me home. When I was in the car I opened the letter from Jay. She had drawn a red flower, and on the back of the picture she had written, 'Love from Jay'.

Chapter Seven
Back to School

When I arrived home from Tadworth Court, I did a tally and realised that I had been off school for a total of seventy-eight days. By the time I went back to Somerford Junior School on Monday 4th March 1968, I was more than ready to meet all my friends and teachers again.

I made my way into the classroom, and took my usual seat. 'Hello, Antony,' said the girl who always sat next to me. 'I kept your seat warm, just like I said I would. But why did you take so long to get back to school? Don't you like me any more?'

'Of course I like you,' I said. 'But now I have got to catch up with my school work, and if you don't mind, little madam, I have got to concentrate'.

I settled back in, and started trying to catch up with the English and Maths that I had missed. After just a few weeks though, it was the Easter Holidays, and although I tried to read and work at home I had lost all confidence in my ability to do the work.

By the time I went back to school after Easter I was really at a very low ebb. I was getting nosebleeds with bad headaches, and I was miserable because I put myself under so much pressure to try to do well. I soon became despondent, because try as I might I could not seem to manage to read, write, spell or do my sums. I had always loved music, but even playing the piano seemed to be beyond my abilities now. I was so embarrassed, and because I failed to make allowances for what I had been through, I began to think of myself as a complete failure.

Eventually I started to read picture books, hoping that these would get me used to reading again. I even tried to read the Sunday newspapers, and to my surprise I found my ability improving. My confidence slowly returned as I realised that I was learning to read all over again.

Now I had to sort out my English and Maths, but that was proved hard. I could count to one hundred very fast indeed, but I had trouble doing my times tables and fractions. I remember that in Art, my favourite subject, I had to make a balsa wood model aeroplane. I found it hard to handle the tools, and when I did finally manage to make the model it would not fly. It landed in the dustbin, and that was where it stayed. Next I was told to make a Gonk, again out of balsa. It looked like me, I thought, as I stared at the finished product.

Things brightened up in October, when I had a wonderful celebration for my tenth birthday, and then a brilliant Christmas to round the year off. I always liked the New Year, with its promise of a fresh start, and this year I tried again to make a big effort to concentrate on my studies at school.

Meanwhile, Dad had bought me a two wheeler bike, called a Pave Master, from Honeybuns, our local bike shop. The idea was to help me exercise my legs. I had never ridden a bike yet before and I loved the freedom of it. I learned to ride quickly, and was soon bombing around the streets with my friends. I was becoming more mobile all the time.

One day I was out cycling with my family. We were

riding down a footpath close to Ashtree Riding School, on the way to Stanpit Marsh. We were approaching a short steep hill, so I pedalled as hard as I could, my little legs spinning at the speed of light to try to reach the top. But I hit a big stone, and went flying off the bike head first into a ditch. I was knocked out for several minutes, but luckily my Mum and Nanny came to the rescue and dragged me out.

I was covered from head to toe in thick horrible mud, and smelled like a compost heap. I had cut my hand badly, and Mum couldn't stop the bleeding, so I was driven to the Royal Victoria Hospital in Boscombe, Bournemouth, to have stitches put in. By then the thick mud had dried up on my clothes and I felt like a cooked mud cake in the clean, sterile surroundings of the hospital.

The doctor who stitched up my hand decided that I should have a mild anti-tetanus injection, as Mum was not sure whether I had had one recently. The injection was administered in my bottom and it really hurt. I had my arm up in a sling for a week after this event. It made me feel like Evel Knievel!

Around that time, my Grandad bought a chestnut horse. He was a beautiful animal, and we named him Ricky, after the American TV programme, 'Champion the Wonder Horse'. I used to be scared of the big horses at Ashtree, because I was so tiny. I was convinced that the huge creatures looming over me were about to gobble me up. But Ricky was special to me from the first.

Most days after school I would head to his stable to fill his net with hay and feed him rolled oats, bran, barley and sugar beet. Then I helped the stable hands to clean the stable, and I'd clean his saddle too. I was given extra pocket money for all this.

The Riding School was becoming busy as it was getting better established. There were a number of members of staff now, working hard behind the scenes. The bookings were flooding in for day treks in the New Forest, and for riding lessons in the evenings in the big floodlit main paddock. There was a pony club, which was great fun to watch – my Uncle Matt would put on show jumping competitions for the club members.

For a distraction from business, Grandad Cook had bought a beautiful long wooden cabin cruiser, with four big port holes on both sides of the bow. On the stern of the boat was a large cabin with a big wheel to steer, a hand cut wooden table, and luxury cushioned seats. The boat was moored on the River Avon.

One day, Grandad and Nanny took Mum, Dad, Julie and I out for a day trip around the Isle of Wight. We all took our fishing rods, and Mum made a picnic hamper for us to eat on board. It was a hot summer's day, and the sea was calm.

We started out from Christchurch Quay, heading towards Mudeford Quay, the main entrance which would take us out to sea. This entrance is called The Run, and it can bring deep fast waters and tricky currents. That day the tide came out against us very fast, and the boat was tossing and turning frantically.

We all held on as tight as we could. 'Albert! Albert!' yelled Nanny Cook. 'I have had enough of this now. I want to go home'.

Grandad didn't answer her. At that point the picnic hamper, which was being tossed around the cabin, came unfastened and its contents spilled out over the cabin and out on deck. To add further confusion, a flock of seagulls bombarded us then, trying to snatch the food from the decking.

Things did improve, and we reached the Isle of Wight, where we decided to stop for a few hours to fish. The sun was boiling hot, and the sea was calm. Nanny smothered herself in suntan cream, put her dark glasses on, and placed a large white headscarf on her head. She lay back to relax, cigarette in mouth, perhaps fancying herself as a 1950's actress on a boat in St Tropez.

Grandad soon spoiled her reverie though, by landing an enormous Tope shark. These are England's most common shark, and this was a really large haul – it took Grandad a huge effort to reel it in. Dad eventually helped him to get it onto the boat – and it was taller than me! Grandad had to put the fish back into the water though, because Nanny refused to let him bring it home.

We moored the boat at Yarmouth, a harbour on the Isle of Wight. We'd lost our picnic to the seagulls, so we had to buy food. There were lots of people on holiday at Yarmouth, which was a nice sight to see, but I soon discovered myself to be the centre of attention. I was embarrassed because people were staring at me and my built up black shoe. I poked my tongue out at the grown-ups, and they stopped staring and went off huffily.

But the children carried on laughing, and calling out to their mothers, 'Look at that boy!'

One boy in particular kept making fun of me, so I kicked his ankle and he cried out in pain. I shouted out, 'It's not so funny now, is it? I hope it hurts you just like you hurt me. Leave me alone now, you big bully, and go and pick on someone your own size'.

The boy's parents were very cross with him for teasing me, and made him apologise. Afterwards, his Dad gave him a clip around the ear and made him cry. I was pleased with the result of my actions – there was one boy who wouldn't be teasing anybody because of their disability again!

On the 21st July 1969 the world seemed to come to a standstill, while many people gathered around television screens to watch Neil Armstrong become the first man to walk on the moon. This was the subject of conversation for days afterwards. It was school summer holidays, but all my friends wanted to talk about was the Moon landing. 'Antony,' my friend said to me over and over, 'Antony, when I grow up I am going to be a spaceman'.

'When I grow up,' I replied. 'I want to be a famous artist and a creative designer'. It was the first time I had voiced this ambition, but my love of art was coming to the fore. I was very good at art, especially at drawing buildings. I had a picture book of buildings that interested me, and I spent hours copying them with HB pencils and biros. Sometimes I used watercolour paints, and drew and painted huge buildings on plain wallpaper lining paper.

I found drawing very relaxing, and it was also great therapy for my fingers, to make them more flexible. I took up playing the piano again, and taught myself a new tune called Greensleeves, which remains my favourite music to this day. I still hadn't learned to read music, but I was able to play by ear.

I was still determined to concentrate on my school work, but the new term was not far in when I had a terrible setback. It was during an English lesson that the pain struck. I had just finished writing some notes, but as I tried to get up out of my chair to give them to the teacher, I realised that I was stuck.

I was crying out in agony – my left hip joint had dislocated. The English teacher, Mr Holloway, came over to my side, looking very concerned, and asking what was the matter.

I started screaming then. 'Help me, Sir!' I shouted. 'Please help me! It hurts so much!'

Everyone was staring in shock. Mr Holloway called for assistance, and two teachers managed to carry me between them to the sick bay, near the Headteacher's office. Suddenly, what sounded to me like a huge bang and crunch came from my hip joint, which had slotted back into place.

Mr Hackett called my parents and they both came to the school to collect me. Mum phoned Dr Cantlie then, who came straight over to check the movement in my leg and hip. I was still in a lot of pain.

The doctor advised that I should not go back to school, in case my hip dislocated again. He rang Dr Lloyd Roberts' secretary at Great Ormond Street and asked for an urgent appointment. I could sense that further upheaval was on its way, just as I had thought things were going to settle down. I felt really upset and confused.

There was no use railing against fate though, and I simply resigned myself to whatever was going to happen next. Just two days later an appointment came in the post, for me to see Mr Lloyd Roberts at Great Ormond Street on September 19th.

I had X-rays taken on both hips, and when I was shown in to see the doctor, he smiled at me. 'These visits are becoming a bit of a habit, Antony,' he said. 'Anyhow, we have looked at the X-rays and found out what has caused the problems with your hips. You have arthritis on both hip joints. As you don't have much joint space and the bone is very rough, the cartilage has worn, and that is what is causing the pain'.

'So what happens now?' I asked.

'Back to Tadworth Court, I'm afraid. We're going to need you to stay there again so that we can do some tests. I would like you to go in October – you will stay on ZMA ward again, for at least nine days. You can bring your bicycle – part of your physiotherapy programme will include riding around the grounds'. He turned to his secretary and began to dictate a letter to her, 'I would like to book Antony Evans into Tadworth Court, ZMA ward, on the 20th October. He will need nine days of hard work on a physio programme'.

Then the doctor spoke to my Mum. 'Before your son goes to Tadworth Court, Mrs Evans, I will ask Dr Cantlie to arrange with the school to give him some homework to do each day, so that he won't fall behind'.

Later that day, at home, Mum and Dad explained to me that there was no need to worry, because this time I would not be having any operations. I would only need the physio programme to help me regain my strength.

So, just after my eleventh birthday, I travelled back to Tadworth Court. I met the same Sister and the same fantastic nurses who had looked after me previously. I even had the same bed and bedside locker as before. There was a nip in the air – chestnut and conker trees were shedding their leaves outside in the wonderful gardens. My bike was unloaded from the car and stored in the corridor entrance, ready for work to begin.

The next morning the physiotherapist arrived at my bedside. She said she would like me to embark on my new exercise programme immediately. 'You can ride your bike around the grounds,' she told me, 'Through the archway paths and back past the main building of Tadworth Court, and then back towards your ward'.

I set off as instructed, riding very slowly because my hip joints were very painful. They felt as though they were cracking, and I began to cry with the pain. I couldn't dismount from the bike because of the agony, but I managed to stop for a rest. Suddenly I felt a bombardment, a barrage of shiny hard things from the sky. I looked up to see what seemed like hundreds of squirrels eating chestnuts in the trees above, throwing the hard shells down onto me.

I went on like this day after day, riding around the grounds. I soon relaxed, and began to feel like the Lord of the Manor as I sailed past Tadworth Court in all its glory several times a day. After some days my hips were getting stronger, and I was in less pain.

At the end of the week, a nurse approached me and said, 'Antony, this time I am going to use a stopwatch to time you. I want you to ride around the grounds and back to your ward as fast as you can – but don't knock any nurses over on the way!'

'Okay,' I agreed. It was a quiet sunny day, very cold, with traces of mist in the air. The trees were shedding leaves in earnest, and I could smell the rich soil of the countryside.

'Are you ready, Antony?' the nurse enquired.

'No,' I said. 'I am bursting for a wee'.

The nurse was clearly frustrated. 'Go on then, if you have to,' she said. 'But get a move on'.

I relieved myself, came back and mounted my bike again, ready for the countdown. 'Are you ready?' the nurse asked again.

'No,' I told her.

'What is it this time?' she groaned.

'I've got a puncture,' I said.

The nurse looked down at my tyres for a moment, bemused, before the penny dropped. 'No you haven't, you cheeky little monkey!' she exclaimed, but I was already pedalling off.

I pedalled away fast, building up speed as I rode through the archways. There was a slope now and I was travelling even faster.   Just as I realised I had forgotten to turn off I sailed straight down the slope into the basement of Tadworth Court.   I stopped quickly, and managed to turn the bike around and head off up the slope before I was challenged.   Hopefully nobody had spotted me in the hospital building on my bike.

When I got back to the nurse she was smiling. 'I must say you have regained a lot of movement in your hips, Antony. Well done! But don't be so cheeky next time, or I will set those squirrels after you again'.

My stay at Tadworth was coming to a close now. One morning I was told to go for a long morning walk to see how I would cope.   I walked around the grounds, wrapped in my thick coat to protect me from the cold air. I came to a building I had never seen before – white with beautiful windows – it reminded me of Ashtree House with its wonderful shuttered windows.

Beneath my feet, lying between the lovely wild flowers on the lawns, were hundreds of conkers and chestnuts. I forgot that I was supposed to be walking as part of my exercise regime, and started to collect these, storing them in my coat pocket. My charge nurse turned up then, with two others. 'So this is where you've been hiding!' she exclaimed. 'I nearly sent out a search party, but here you are collecting chestnuts and conkers. You're supposed to be out walking!' The other nurses could not contain their laughter.

I spoke to my nurse. 'I just wanted them to give to my friends when I go home!'
She took me back to the ward then, and helped me to store all my goodies in a bedpan, to keep them fresh.

Later that evening, the sister called me to her office. 'I've heard you have been giving my nurses a hard time, Antony,' she said, with a twinkle in her eye. 'I am very proud of you, you have worked very hard on your Physio programme and made excellent progress. Your Mum and Dad will be coming to take you home tomorrow. You can return to school, and Mr Lloyd Roberts will send an appointment for you to attend Great Ormond Street early next year'.

The next day Mum and Dad arrived, both very pleased to see me moving so much more easily. I was happy to see them too, of course, but I felt sad to leave Tadworth Court, where I had been so well looked after and had so much fun. Without the shadow of an operation looming over me, my stay had really seemed more like a holiday than anything else. I hadn't even been homesick, this time.

'Thank you for having me,' I called out to all the nurses as I left. 'Goodbye!'

I set my sights forward then. It was my final year at the Juniors, and I knew I had to focus now to keep up with the others. All the teachers were good to me, and tried hard to help my in my endeavours. But I gradually became very low in mood – I convinced myself that I was just not capable, no matter how hard I tried to apply myself to the school work. Soon I lost interest in everything and everybody, and just wanted to stay at home in my room.

My Mum and Dad were very concerned. They could see I was stressed and upset and they didn't know what to do when I refused to go to school. I regressed physically too – the bed was wet every morning when I woke up, because I had developed such a fear of school.

I just wanted to be normal like everybody else, and to learn at school with all my friends – but somehow I had completely lost my confidence. I started to feel very isolated and lonely. Times were hard.

Julie was in her last year of Twynham Comprehensive School now, and was working hard ready for her move to Brockenhurst College (in the New Forest) in September. One day Julie had left her homework on the kitchen table and I took a quick peep. I was amazed to see her beautiful handwriting, neat and tidy just like my Mum's.

I was inspired by this, and decided that I would like to go to Twynham too. Mum and I went to see the headteacher there, Mr Cotton, and we both liked him immediately - he was a tall man, very kind and with a cheerful manner.

Mum explained to Mr Cotton about my disabilities and how long periods in hospital had made me behind with my school work, and he seemed to understand.

And that was it – I was in!

I did feel sad to say goodbye to all my teachers and friends from the Junior School though. My music teacher, Mrs Tickner, asked me to come to the school hall with her and play 'Les Petites Enfants' on the grand piano there. She gave me a big hug when she had finished.

'This tune will always make me think of you,' she said.

Chapter Eight
Secondary School

On Wednesday 9th September 1970, when I was nearly twelve years old, I started at Twynham Comprehensive School. It wasn't easy during my first week - I had a lot of walking to do, to make my way between the classrooms for each different subject, and it felt as though I was trying to find my way through a maze. Sometimes I did get lost, but somehow eventually I became used to it all.

The second week was even worse. I had to carry all my text books and library books around the school in my brief case, and they were very heavy. I felt self-conscious too, because I was such a small boy with tiny hands and huge built up shoes. But everyone seemed to be able to look deeper than my surface appearance, and they accepted me for who I was. I soon settled in, and made a good start.

Lessons varied from half an hour to one hour in length. I took General Science, Geography, Music, Art, Mathematics, English, Religious Education and History. I was only interested in a few of these though – Art, Music, Science, History and Geography. As far as I was concerned, the others could be disregarded – I paid them no attention whatsoever.

I did want to do PE though. I loved playing football, and I asked the teacher whether I could join in with the other boys on the football pitch. He was sympathetic, but said he would have to ask the Headteacher, because he was not sure about whether I would be able to wear football boots.

After consulting my mother, Mr Cotton agreed that yes, I could play football. He looked at me seriously though. 'You do realise that if you have any problems with your legs, you must stop immediately,' he told me, and I promised to do so.

I was delighted to find that I turned out to be quite good at football. While I was playing I would pretend that I was the world-famous Brazilian footballer Pele. I am a great supporter of Brazil. In June 1970, the summer before I started at Twynham, the World Cup had been held in Mexico. To my delight, Brazil had played Italy in the final and won the match, by four goals to one.

One morning, the headteacher announced that each and every one of us would be taking part in a ten mile sponsored walk from Twynham School to Boscombe Pier and back again. The idea was to raise enough money to build a roof for the school swimming pool.

I was very excited when I got home, and immediately gave the details of the sponsored walk to my mother. She glanced at the sheets, then looked at me. 'You do realise, Antony, that there is no question of you taking part. With your disabilities, it would be a physical impossibility to walk ten miles'.

'I'm sure I can do it, Mum,' I said. 'I know I can. Please let me take part'.

Eventually my parents agreed that I could try, and I was delighted. I went round to visit all my neighbours, and the families of my friends, and asked them to sponsor me. When the day finally arrived, the weather was perfect – warm and sunny. We all arrived at school wearing our uniforms, ready to start. I was very excited, although a little nervous.

Twynham School had clearly put a lot of time and effort into planning this sponsored walk. They gave us detailed instructions regarding the route – there was no excuse for anyone to get lost, or to take a short cut! In fact, there were various checkpoints stationed all along the way, manned by members of staff. There were also very strict guidelines as to the behaviour expected from us while we were walking.

I was just about to set off on the walk when Mr Cotton approached me. 'I still can't quite believe you are going ahead with this,' he said. 'It's not too late to change your mind'.

I shook my head. 'No, Sir!' I said. 'No one is going to stop me. But if you are going to be waiting here, you might need your camp bed'.

He didn't know what to say to that, so I started walking right then. Setting off through the streets on my ten mile journey it all felt quite easy at first. I was soon signing at the checkpoint for my first mile. Then I walked down a path to Southbourne Promenade, where we continued, the sand and sea to our left as we strode along. I was keeping up with all the others, and my legs felt fine, although the weather seemed to be getting hotter by the minute.

Mum was walking alongside me, and Dad was driving his car on the road which runs on the cliff top above the beach. Dad had his binoculars, so he could keep an eye out in case it all got too much for me. It was such a fine day that all the occupants of the beach huts were out in force, cheering us on. One man shouted at me, 'Go on, son, you can do it! Good luck!'

I was heading towards my third check point, cruising along very nicely. The teachers kept asking if I was okay, and whether I would like to sit down. I just smiled at them and kept going. I sensed that if I sat, even for a short time, my legs would stiffen and I would not be able to carry on. Mum was walking behind me now, and she started to feel quite concerned, but she said nothing because she knew how much it meant to me to join in with the other children, and prove that I could do just the same as them.

When the walkers reached the half way mark at Boscombe beach, my house tutor was waiting. He looked astounded to see me. 'This is fantastic!' he said, 'Fantastic!'

All the other teachers seemed equally impressed. I knew I had another five miles to go, but I was encouraged by all the people who kept coming up to me and patting me on my shoulder to wish me luck.

I set off again. In the pocket of my school trousers I had hundreds of Smarties in case I got hungry. But hunger was the least of my worries. The heat was building and really starting to bother me now. It was a wonderful day – the sky was blue and the beach was filled with people lying on the sand or in their deckchairs. Some of the men had their heads covered with handkerchiefs to protect their scalps from the sun.

It all looked idyllic – but these were far from ideal walking conditions. Apart from the searing heat, there were large crowds of people on the promenade, which made progress difficult. But on we pressed, back the same route we had come. This was becoming hard work now – and when I looked at my watch I saw it was already three o'clock. I was still trying to keep up with the other children but as we passed the six mile checkpoint I was being overtaken by more and more of them, and slowly drifting behind.

'Keep going, Antony,' my friends urged me as they passed. 'You can do it – don't give up!'

I glanced behind me then, and saw another group of children coming up behind me at what seemed like a great speed. I started to feel despondent. I was very tired now, and had cramp in my legs and blisters on my feet, caused by wearing my surgical shoes all day. My school shirt was soaked with the perspiration pouring down my face and back.

Mum looked at me. 'You need to stop, son,' she said gently. 'Call it a day now'.

'I am not giving up,' I told her. 'I don't care if it takes me until midnight – I am going to finish this walk'.

I couldn't help slowing down, though. It was half past four. My back and ribs were hurting, and I found it hard to keep walking in a straight line. I had reached Tuckton bridge now, and I knew it wasn't far to the school, but I had to hold on to the railing for support. I felt close to collapse.

My body was trying to tell me to stop, that I had overreached the limit of what it could bear. I ignored it, because I was so determined to finish the walk, although I had tears streaming down my face from the pain. It was all a huge effort, but as I finally crossed the bridge I could see the school finish line, and struggled on towards it.

I put on a brave face, and mustered all the strength I had to reach that line. Some of the waiting teachers and children began to cheer me on. The distance grew smaller – fifty yards to go – twenty – ten – and then at last I was there, and threw myself exhausted over the finish line.

The applause began, and seemed as though it would last forever. One of the teachers picked me up and shouted out, 'For Antony's a jolly good fellow!' and the others all sang out, 'Hip, hip, hooray!' in response.

I finally sat down, and watched my tutor sign the card to confirm that I had finished the ten mile walk. Mr Cotton looked down at me. 'I will never forget what you have done today, Antony,' he said. 'Thank you for being such a kind, brave boy. Well done you!'

Now that I had stopped walking, my strength quickly began to return. Dad was waiting to take me home, and I climbed into the car and lay stretched out on the back seat. I had stiffened up by the time we reached our house, and Mum gave me a comforting cup of tea, and cooked a hot meal.

The next morning was Saturday. It was pouring with rain, so my friend Garry, who lived nearby, invited me around to play with his Airfix soldiers and tanks. Garry and I played together regularly on rainy days, scattering toy soldiers all around the table and chairs in his lounge, inventing our own war games.

To make things fair, both of us had a small eighth army

gun, which we loaded with caps and matchsticks. When we let go of the gun pin, the caps made a mighty bang, and the matchsticks shot out of the barrels to knock down the opposing army's soldiers. I didn't mind the rain – I enjoyed the war games as much as I did the football.

Most weekends though I spent a lot of time alone, playing with my collection of Corgi, Dinky and Match Box Super Fast cars. I was quite happy with my own company. I was delighted, though, when the family got a puppy – a poodle – at the end of November. Pickles the Poodle had a long pedigree, and his Kennel Club name was Laughing Cavalier. It was an apt name too - he had a grin just like Dennis the Menace's dog, Gnasher.

Pickles was supposed to be an apricot colour, but as the weeks passed he turned out to be patchy in colour – black and white mixed with the apricot. The breeder was aghast and offered to take him back, but of course by then we had all fallen in love with him and there was no way we could part with him.

Pickles was a real character. He loved playing games – his favourite was Hunt the Chocolate Drops. He was very well trained – eventually we only needed to point to the door for him to wait outside until he was called in. He would become bored if he was left outside for too long though, and then he would peep around the door, or even tap on it.

He loved seeing the beautician and got very excited when she called to collect him. When he returned, shampooed and perfumed, he was not so happy, and used to sulk under a chair until we managed to coax him out. 'Look what a sight they have made out of me!' he seemed to be thinking.

Pickles knew when his bedtime was – and at exactly ten o'clock each night he would perform what we called his 'War Dance' to show us he was now ready to go to sleep. He was my best friend, and my parents even wondered whether he should visit Great Ormond Street with me, as we turned out to have similar hip problems!

Chapter Nine
Music

I still liked to play the piano, and around that time one of my oldest friends, Nigel, who lived nearby, taught me how to play the cornet, a beautiful brass musical instrument. I loved it, and when I told my Grandad about it, he offered to buy one for me. I asked Mr Wilson, the music teacher at Twynham, whether I could have music lessons.

'Of course you can, Antony,' he said. 'But we only play trumpets at school, not cornets'.

I told Grandad that Mr Wilson would be pleased to give me trumpet lessons at school, starting as soon as I wished, and he took me to Eddie Moors music shop in Boscombe to buy a trumpet. When we entered the shop I was amazed to see such a huge variety of classical instruments – violins, drum sets, cellos, guitars, flutes, grand pianos, french horns and many more.

Eddie Moors was a friend of my Grandad, and they stood chatting together while I looked around. The trumpets all cost over a hundred pounds, and I felt a bit embarrassed by the prices. 'Have you seen the trumpet you want, Antony?' asked my Grandad. 'I have,' I said, 'But it's far too expensive.'

'Which one do you like?' asked my Grandad.

'This one,' I said. 'It's a Jupiter trumpet with a three valve, and a lacquer yellow brass body'.

The shop owner took the instrument out of the display case and let me hold it. I started to play a scale, up and down. It had a rich tone and felt just the right size – there was no pain in my fingers as I held it. It was a very impressive instrument. Even the case looked posh – made of black leather with red velvet material inside.

I was proud to take my trumpet to my first lesson at school the next day. I had to play from a Gatti Duet book for trumpets. I could read the music quite easily and the teacher, who was impressed, asked me to take an early exam.

The exam was to be held at a boys' school in Winchester, and I was very excited. However, when the day of the exam came I was horrendously nervous, messed up because of my nerves and failed the exam. I was already struggling a bit with the trumpet. My arms ached with the effort of holding it up when I played, and when the trumpet was in its case I could hardly carry it around.

I confided in my Grandad, who told me not to worry. 'We'll take it back to Eddie Moors,' he said, 'And exchange it for something smaller'. Mr Wilson, the music teacher, suggested that I have a cornet after all. He said my music book could be used for cornets as well as trumpets.

When Grandad and I went to the shop we were met again by Eddie Moor, who showed me a cornet. It was beautifully made, and so was its case. The price tag was over four hundred pounds. 'Is it an English make, Mr Moor?' I asked.

'No,' he said. 'This cornet was made in Austria, for the top young musicians there to learn to play classical music on'. The instrument was a blend of gold, yellow and silver, and it was so shiny that it reflected back like a mirror. When I played it, it sounded even better than the trumpet, and it was a lot easier to use. My arms and fingers no longer ached, and I was very happy.

That year I got lots of records for Christmas presents. I was very fond of music and I loved classical and film themes. My favourite movie soundtrack was Born Free, sung by Matt Munro. It still has the power to move me to tears sometimes.

It was Pickles the Poodle's first Christmas with our family. He liked helping us unwrap our presents. He used to take one end of the paper in his mouth and tug as hard as he could, getting tangled up in a bundle of sticky Sellotape as a result, and thoroughly enjoying every minute of the fun. There was lots of chocolate around at this time of year - Pickles loved the smell of chocolate. He was great to have around, and made our family Christmas even more enjoyable than usual!

The Christmas holidays had not begun well, though. At the start of the holidays, Mum had asked me whether I'd received a school report for my first term at Twynham.

'No,' I replied innocently. 'Perhaps the school forgot to give me one'.

Later that day, Mum appeared, brandishing my school report, 'Look what I found under your bed, young man. I think you have some explaining to do!' she said sternly.

My head went down and I flushed bright red. 'I'm so sorry, Mum,' I said. 'I have been finding it hard to do my school work, and I didn't want you to be disappointed in me. And I was scared in case you told me off'.

'I've looked at the report,' she said. 'And it isn't that bad. You have done very well with your General Science, Music, Art, Geography and R.E. I know you find Maths and English hard, but that's okay'.

'The pain is stopping me from learning again,' I told her. 'It hurts so much that I can't concentrate'.

'I only want you to do your best,' said my Mum. 'I don't mind what marks you get, as long as you keep trying'.

'I just want to be normal, like everyone else at school,' I told her, and I knew she understood.

I made my usual New Year's resolutions: to do better at school, to listen more and to work harder at reading and writing. Even as I resolved to do my best, I sensed that the year ahead would not be an academic success.

As soon as I arrived back at school in January, my English teacher started to hassle me. She was convinced that if I tried harder I could produce better work. She nagged at me so much that I felt I was being victimised, but I didn't want to report it in case this made matters worse. I decided to wait and see what happened.

I didn't have too long to wait. One day the English teacher took our whole class on a trip to Lulworth Cove. She let some of the class smoke cigarettes at Lulworth, although she was in clear contradiction of the school rules by doing so. She also allowed us to wander off alone, although we should have been supervised. We nearly came to a sticky end this way – we all raced to the top of a hill, and then almost toppled into the sea –

we were right on the edge of the cliff. Fortunately, everybody managed to stop just in time.

When I got home later, I told my Mum what had happened. She was very worried and upset. Next morning Mr Cotton called me to his office. 'Your mother has told me some disturbing news about your school trip, Antony,' he said. 'Is this true?'

'Yes, Sir,' I said, and then I told him about how the teacher had been bullying me. Apparently there had been other complaints about her, and consequently the school board gave her an official warning.

Around that time my neighbour's friend, Mr Farge, asked whether I would like to join the Bournemouth Silver Band, playing my cornet. Rehearsals were held every Wednesday night in Bournemouth. I was delighted with the invitation, and accepted immediately.

The next day at school I told Mr Wilson that I was going to join the Bournemouth Silver Band. 'That's amazing, Antony,' he said. 'I'm so pleased you didn't let the incident with your trumpet exam put you off music altogether'.

At my first rehearsal I met the band conductor, who welcomed me to the band. 'I hear you have a new cornet,' he said. 'Could I have a look?'

When he saw the cornet, his eyes brightened immediately. 'What a wonderful instrument,' he said. 'It's beautiful, fantastic. One of the top cornets, made in Austria'.

I then introduced myself to a lady who stood nearby.

'Hello,' I said, 'My name is Antony. Who are you?'

'I'm Midge,' she said. 'Hi. I'll look after you if you get stuck on the high notes.'

'How many are there in the band?' I asked, and she told me that there were about thirty-five members.

By now all the seats were laid out, with music sheets on music stands. The band members filtered into the hall slowly with their instruments – cornets, trombones, euphoniums, tubas, drums and percussion. I realised with a shock that they were nearly all old men – Midge was the only female in the group and I was the only boy. All the instruments they were about to play looked ancient and beaten up – I felt like I had joined a Dad's Army band!

The conductor announced that we were going to play Oklahoma, and we tuned our instruments. The conductor counted, one, two and three... and bang on cue the huge drum with cymbals attached collapsed and crashed down in a noisy, tuneless heap onto the floor.

I couldn't help laughing, although I felt sorry for the poor old man in charge of the drum. After fifteen minutes he sorted himself out, and we started to play Oklahoma. It was not good – the tempo kept shifting from fast to slow and back again. Old Man River came out even worse. It took the whole evening to rehearse these two songs. I was bored stiff, and very relieved when the evening came to an end.

The conductor came over to me as the band were packing up to leave. 'I was watching you,' he said. 'You looked very puzzled when we played Old Man River'.

'I don't like to be rude,' I said, 'But that music is way too old fashioned. We should play something from the sixties and seventies musicals. Like West Side Story, the Sound of Music, South Pacific, The King and I – just to name a few'.

The conductor said that he would give it some thought, and in the Spring when we had a meeting about the forthcoming Summer Season Concert, he announced that we would include some of these songs.

Meanwhile I took my Year One school exams, and I was delighted that I passed each one, albeit with low grades. July 23rd was the last day of the summer term, and the day our reports came out. The best thing was that there was no need to try to hide it from my Mum this time!

The Bournemouth Silver Band Summer Season Concert was held in Fisherman's Walk, at the Bandstand, on a Saturday afternoon in the school holidays. We had a large audience - there were hundreds of deckchairs set up, each occupied by pensioners who all seemed to have brought picnics. The mood was very much, 'Last Night of the Proms' – or rather, 'The Last Afternoon of the Proms'.

We opened by playing, 'The Sound of Music', which went down a treat. We followed up with 'West Side Story'. Then one of the band members went around with a collection box to raise funds. After the break, we played 'Paint Your Wagon' and Lee Marvin's famous song 'Wandering Star', and the old people joined in, singing slowly in time with the band. I was amazed that they remembered all the words!

The band was getting stronger now that it had an influx of new fresh ideas. We wore a uniform – black trousers, black jacket, a white shirt and a long blue tie. I didn't need to buy anything new, because my school uniform was almost exactly the same design! I continued to attend band practice every Wednesday evening, and began to settle properly into the band. I made plenty of friends there, although I was the youngest by far.

The summer was nearly over, and one afternoon Mum and Dad announced that they had a surprise. Soon a van arrived, and out of it came our first colour television – truly a momentous event!

Back in school in September, there was a strong emphasis on metalwork and woodwork. I made an aluminium ladle in metalwork, and thought it was not a bad effort, although it was a little shallow. However, the metalwork teacher looked at my handiwork disparagingly, and laughed in a not-unfriendly manner.

'Antony,' he said, 'I think it would take at least twenty goes to fill a soup bowl with that ladle.

I looked at him, and said nothing. What I was thinking was, 'If you don't stop giggling, I will shove the soup bowl over your head!' But I didn't have a soup bowl (or any soup) and anyway I wouldn't have been tall enough to reach, so my violent imaginings came to nothing.

I didn't fare any better at woodwork. My heart sank the first time I entered the woodwork room – I could see at a glance that the benches would be too tall for me to reach. The teacher was helpful, making a long wooden step for me to stand on. We were all supplied with basic hand tools and the teacher asked the class to each make a wooden coat peg. I drew a plan of my peg, and showed it to the teacher, who was impressed. 'Good luck,' he said. 'I hope it turns out well'.

I started to measure the peg stem and base. That went well, but using the handsaw to cut out the pieces of wood was a nightmare. I found it hard to grip the handsaw, and my hand became sweaty, and soon began to blister. It was extremely painful.

I carried on though, making a small square joint on one end of the peg and a square hole joint in the middle of the base, by using a small wooden chisel and a wooden mallet. The mallet was very heavy, and every time I tried to bang the chisel with the mallet to make a hole on the base, the bones in my arms felt as though they were cracking. By the time I had finished, my fingers looked like a set of Wall's sausages, but on the bright side I had made my first coat peg.

I handed the coat peg and plan drawing to the woodwork teacher for marking, and sat back down at my desk to await his comments. It wasn't long before he made his way over, and stood for a while, looking down at me. Suddenly he burst out laughing.

'Well,' said the teacher, 'I have never seen anything quite like this before. This coat peg is upside down, and it is covered in thick wooden glue. It is a great effort though, and I will give you 45% for trying so hard'.

I wasn't the only one struggling with woodwork – none of my friends seemed to find it easy either. Clearly, neither metalwork or woodwork were going to be my strong points in life – although I did think the coat peg might have made a nice exhibit in the Tate Modern

Gallery in London. People could have travelled from far and wide to marvel at it, and wonder what it was. And the ladle might not have been much practical use – but it has lasted well, for I still have it to this day!

Another big event was approaching for the Bournemouth Silver Band – we were due to perform a Christmas Concert in Bournemouth. I made sure to practice my cornet frequently at home around that time – I had never played live on stage before, and so I was a little anxious.

There were hundreds of people queuing up outside the Playhouse Theatre when we arrived that evening. Mum and Dad dropped me off at the stage door and went around to join the long queue at the front. The band were all equally nervous, and before we went on stage we braced ourselves mentally to face the huge crowd.

We started to play, and the curtain reeled up. To our astonishment the auditorium was almost empty – only about twenty people filled the five hundred seat theatre. We carried on, feeling as though we were engaged in band practice rather than a performance. During the interval the conductor came to speak to us. 'I'm so sorry about the size of the audience,' he said. 'The queues outside were not for us, I'm afraid. All those people were queuing for the Galaxy Cinema next door'.

Some of the band members took this personally, packed up their instruments and left. The conductor asked the rest of us to vote on whether we wanted to postpone the second half of the show. Midge and I voted to carry on, and that turned out to be the majority view, although we knew it would be hard now that we had lost some of our most experienced players.

We changed the stage set so that it suited a twelve piece band, and when the curtain reel went up for a second time we began to play, 'I'm Dreaming of a White Christmas'. Gradually, there was an influx of more people into the theatre, who started to join in with the song. Next we played, 'We Wish you a Merry Christmas'. This was a smart call – the atmosphere began to improve, the audience began to cheer and shout out, 'More! More!'

We were all delighted and relieved - the audience stayed enthralled in their seats right up to the end of the concert. I was worn out by the end of it all, but buoyed up by the fuss that Mum and Dad made of me.

Later that week, I had my last band practice of the year. At the end of it, Midge handed me a brown envelope. 'Don't spend it all at once, Antony,' she advised.

When I opened the envelope, I found to my surprise fifteen pounds nestling inside. 'Wow! What have I done to deserve this, Midge?' I asked.

'At the end of the Bournemouth Silver Band season we share out the collection box takings,' she told me.

I was delighted. This was worth more than ten weeks' pocket money! I had never had so much money before, and I couldn't wait to tell my Mum and Dad.

On the 21st December 1971, I received my Autumn school report. I was disappointed, because my grades had dropped from the previous term. Here are samples of the comments on my report:

English – 'He tries hard, but he forgets to finish all his English homework in time for marking'.

Geography – 'Antony is very slow and wastes much time chattering. His drawing ability is good but his handwriting must improve'.

History – All through, the standard achieved is not high, but he has tried'.

R.E – 'Antony has not done his best this term. He chatters too much. 'Stickability' required'.

On reflection, I think I must have been putting more effort into playing my cornet than I was making with my school work!

It was Christmas time again. Uncle Matt bought me a new USA Spider bike, very similar to the Raleigh Chopper bike. Most of my friends had Raleigh Choppers, but I couldn't ride on one because the seat was too high for me.

My Spider bike had a three speed gear lever attached to the front of the frame. The handle bars were tall and wide, shaped like cow horns. The saddle was low, with a tall back rest. I could get on and off easily. The back wheel was tall and wide with a thick tread. The front wheel was the same size, but without the thick tread.

The gear lever had a 'T' grip shape, and the gear numbers showed inside the three speed panel. The bike was a golden yellow, but the tyres were black and white with wide silver mudguards.

The Raleigh chopper was a cool bike, and the kids that

rode these around had a good deal of street credibility. I was pleased with my bike – it may not have been exactly the same as the others but it had great style of its own.

Later in the day, Grandad held his usual Christmas party at Ashtree House. We had a brilliant time – even Pickles the dog put on a show, fighting with my Nanny's dog Teddy over a Christmas cracker.

Chapter Ten
Fund-Raising

Early in 1972, I became involved with fund-raising for the Guide Dogs for the Blind. I decided I wanted to raise enough money to buy a guide dog. When I broke the news of my latest great idea to my Mum (who was quite pleased that I didn't want to take part in another sponsored walk!) she promised to find out how I would go about doing this.

A few weeks later, Mum announced that she had some good news. 'I have heard from Mr Jones, who has been in touch with the Guide Dog for the Blind Association, and they have agreed that you can buy a dog. It will cost a lot though – two hundred and fifty pounds!'

£250 was an awful lot of money. I was quite taken aback – I realised I would need to organise a lot of events to raise that amount. Despite my misgivings, I soon got stuck in, asking a friend if he would help me to go out to collect jumble. Dad made me a small wooden trailer, designed so that it could be attached to my Spider bike.

My friend and I then went from house to house, asking for jumble. People were very generous and we collected a lot, storing it in my Dad's garage, which soon filled up. We held the jumble sale in the Easter holidays, in my Grandad's front garden. It was on a Saturday, and when I opened the gate hundreds of people stampeded through, leaving me stuck between the gate and the garden wall. I was glad to escape with my life!

I had organised one friend to sell clothes and handbags, another to sell books and comics and a third to sell bric a brac. Mum, Dad, Julie, Nanny and Grandad were in charge of the tea and cakes. Southern Television filmed me and the local paper, the Christchurch Times, did a feature with a photo of me and everyone who had helped.

The whole thing was a great success. The only cloud on the horizon was that even though prices were fixed very low, between two pence and twenty pence per item, many people stole items. I found this petty theft very upsetting – especially because people seemed to be quite brazen about it, tucking things into their pockets and bags quite openly.

The newspaper ran a feature about this, with the headline PILFERING. It was enough to make you lose your faith in human nature, especially since all the proceeds from the sale were to go to charity.

When I counted up the proceeds from the jumble sale, I had made more than forty pounds. I was delighted, and put the whole amount straight into my charity bank account. I realised that I still had a long way to go though.

Meanwhile, I was invited to visit the Guide Dog training centre in Exeter, run by Guide Dogs for the Blind. It was a wonderful place, and I found it very interesting to watch as the animals were trained. The Training Centre bred Labradors, and and raised them until they were ready for training. The Golden Labrador was my favourite breed, although sometimes the charity used black Labradors too. The Golden Labradors seemed to have a great sense of humour, and brilliant shiny golden furry coats. I decided that when I had reached my target of two hundred and fifty pounds, that would be the type of dog I would buy.

After my visit to Exeter I got my thinking cap on, trying to work out some new ideas for fund raising events. Uncle Matt had a brainwave – 'How about a special show jumping event?' he suggested. 'Antony's Charity Challenge Cup, held at Ashtree Riding School Gymkhana?'

'Wow, that would be great!' I said. 'How soon can we do it?'

'I think June would be good,' my uncle replied. 'That will give us some time to organise things. We can invite other riding schools from the New Forest to take part. Hopefully we can raise a lot of money towards your guide dog'.

Back at school, I was still trying to work hard. I found that my least favourite subject was religion, primarily because I don't believe in God or the Bible (I do believe in a Higher Power of some kind, but I find organised religion disappointing).

Mrs Watson, who taught Religious Education, was a very nice lady, and was puzzled by why I never paid attention when she talked about Jesus and his Disciples. One afternoon, she asked each of us in turn whether we believed in God. When it was my turn, she asked me to stand up in front of the class to speak out about my beliefs. 'Okay, Mrs Watson,' I thought to myself, 'You asked, so I will tell you. But you won't like it'.

'I don't believe in God,' I said. 'Jesus was supposed to heal the sick,' I said. 'He touched a blind man's eyes to make him see again. So why did God give newborn children terrible diseases, like my Morquio's Disease? I saw a lot of terrible things when I was at Great Ormond Street, and I don't believe in a God who could make people suffer like that'.

Mrs Watson was very upset. She turned and walked out of the room, leaving me and the rest of the class in silence. After a few minutes another teacher came in, and announced that the class was over.

All the students started to file out of the classroom, but I was asked to stay behind. Apparently, the deputy headteacher, needed to talk to me urgently. So I sat down and waited nervously. I thought I was sure to be punished, but did not know how.

When the deputy head finally arrived, his tone was gentle. 'Mrs Watson is very sorry that she upset you,' he told me. 'She feels that she made a big mistake asking you in front of the whole class whether you believed in God. I am deeply sorry too'.

'Please don't worry, Sir,' I said. 'I'm fine. I was delighted to answer Mrs Watson's question and I'm happy to carry on with religious studies, as long as she is happy to accept that I do not believe in God'.

Later that day, Mrs Watson sought me out. 'Thank you,' she said, and kissed my cheek. 'I used to teach your sister Julie,' she said. 'How is she getting on at Brockenhurst College?'

'Very well, thank you Ma'am,' I answered. And that was that.

One day in an Art lesson Mr Phillips, the teacher, said,

'Antony, I would like you to try pottery. Your task is to make something out of clay, related to sunlight and shadows'.

'Do you mean Cliff Richard and the Shadows, Sir?' I asked, smirking.

'Ha, ha, very funny,' responded Mr Phillips.

I had never done pottery before and had no idea where to start. I looked through a lot of books for inspiration, and eventually found a picture of Stonehenge, which inspired me. I thought about Stonehenge as an ancient temple for worshipping the sun, and imagined the bright morning sunlight shining through the stones, their shadows looming behind.

When I showed my design to the teacher and told him about my ideas, he was very interested. 'I am fascinated to see how your Stonehenge will turn out,' he said.

When I'd finished my model, I gave it to Mr Phillips to put in the kiln. 'Good grief,' he said, 'Your Stonehenge weighs a ton. I hope it doesn't break up when it comes out'. I was worried about this possibility, but it was time to go home, so I'd have to wait until the following day to find out whether Stonehenge had survived its firing.

I walked to Christchurch High Street to catch the bus as usual, and was waiting at the bus stop when I suddenly felt sharp pains shooting down my leg. Looking down, I could see that my knee had swollen. There was quite a long queue of people waiting for the bus, and when I finally got on, it was packed. There was standing room only, so I braced myself to stand and hold onto a rail.

The bus conductor approached me. 'Sorry, son,' he said. 'There are too many people on this bus. You will have to get off and wait for the next one'.

I was in so much pain that it was very difficult to dismount from the bus. The bus conductor made no attempt to help, but just said, 'Hurry up, we're running late'.

I got off the bus feeling very lonely and sad. It was very late now, and I had no idea when the next bus would arrive because the timetable attached to the bus stop had been vandalised.

Mum and Dad arrived at the bus stop looking for me just as I was beginning to get very stressed and upset, and they took me straight home. I told my Mum what had happened, and how my knee still hurt. She decided to arrange for someone to pick me up from school each day, to spare me the strain and struggle of the bus journey.

The swelling and pain from the knee began to subside, but that evening Mum took me to Dr Cantlie for a check-up. He was concerned about my symptoms and worried that my femur might be starting to grow again. He told Mum to keep an eye on things.

The next day I was feeling much better, and was looking forward to finishing off my Stonehenge model. When I got to the Art class, Mr Phillips told me that the model had come out of the kiln intact and was ready to be painted. I used green for the outside of the model, and light brown for the inside, and I chose paintbrushes that were very pointed and smooth, so that I could create special patterns with them. I was very happy, painting and blending the colours and then, when the teacher put the model back into the kiln for its final firing, I went off to my other lessons. The pain in my knee crept back, but I mentioned it to nobody – I didn't want to complain.

Soon it was time for lunch. I queued up with the others and gave my lunch ticket to the prefect in charge. I chose a hot meal from the menu and put it on my tray. Holding the tray, I looked for a place to sit down – but suddenly my knee gave way and I lost control and fell over.

My dinner was all over the floor, and I was crying in pain, but most of the other children were laughing at me. Two teachers came rushing to my side, and the children who were laughing were sent straight to the Head's office. I was taken off to the sick bay, where Mr Cotton came to visit me.

'I have called your parents, Antony,' he said, 'And they are on their way to collect you. I am so sorry for the behaviour of those children'.

'Don't worry about me, Sir,' I said. 'As my Mum always says, sticks and stones may break my bones, but words will never hurt me'.

Mr Cotton smiled. 'You're such a brave little boy,' he said.

Mum took me back to Dr Cantlie, who was very concerned. 'I have heard from your headteacher about your fall, Antony,' he said. 'He also says that you play football at school, and I am afraid that this cannot continue. You can no longer take part in PE lessons'.

I was devastated to hear this. 'But I love playing football! I like doing PE with the rest of my class!'

'Let me explain something to you,' said the doctor. 'If you carry doing PE, you could break your bones and end up in hospital for a very long time. You are already in a lot of pain, I'm sure you don't want it to get worse. And you must put those football boots away. They could cause problems with your hip joints. You have to wear your surgical shoes to keep you properly balanced. That is the reason why you have been fitted with a built up shoe. And meanwhile, we have to keep an eye on that knee of yours'.

Dr Cantlie kept looking at me. 'Do you know,' he said, 'I think you have grown since I last saw you'. He measured me then, and was amazed that I had grown three inches, and was now four feet and seven inches. He thought that I was in pain was because I was still growing – the femur on my bad leg was getting larger.

The doctor had told me to stay off school for a while, to rest my knee. I was soon very bored, and it was a relief when my leg felt much better after a couple of days, and I was allowed to return to school. The first lesson of the day was Art, and as soon as I arrived in the Art room I could see my model of Stonehenge, displayed in a glass cabinet. I was very proud – it looked brilliant!

Mr Phillips came over. 'I must congratulate you on such an unusual piece of art, Antony,' he said. 'I hope you have got somebody to help you take it home, though – it weighs a ton!'

'It's supposed to be heavy, Sir,' I said. 'Stonehenge is made out of stone, which is extremely heavy'. He looked a bit puzzled about that, although it made perfect sense to me!

Later that day, I told the PE teacher what Dr Cantlie had said. 'I'm sorry I won't be seeing you playing football any more,' he replied. 'You play like a Brazilian!' To me, that was the highest praise imaginable.

It was June now, and I was getting very excited about the prospect of the gymkhana at the Ashtree House, to raise some more money for the guide dog.

Uncle Matt had invited a lot of contestants, and my neighbour, Mr Atkins, gave me a special cup to give the winner of my special show jumping event. I called this event 'Antony's Charity Challenge Cup'.

It was a hot, sunny day and the gymkhana was very well organised. The riders were all smartly dressed, and some of the women wore hair nets to keep their hair in place while they were competing, which made them look very posh. The horses all looked immaculately groomed, with lovely shiny coats.

Hundreds of people turned up to watch the show jumping event. An announcement came on over the PA system. 'Good morning ladies and gentlemen. Welcome to Antony's Charity Challenge Cup show jumping event. All the money raised today will go to help Antony Evans to raise funds to buy a Guide Dog for the Blind'.

Over sixty people took part in the event. I handed out the rosettes for first, second and third place, and gave the cup to the winner. We had raised a total of £80. I now had £120 in my special charity bank account, to go towards buying my guide dog.

In July I received the Summer Term school results, and again I was pleased with them. In the holidays the Band Summer Concerts were approaching, and I continued to attend band practice on Wednesday evenings, but there was some discord between the band members and the conductor. The conductor wanted to change the music back to Oklahoma and Show Boat, which was a silly thing to do, and proved to be the catalyst for Midge and many other members to leave the band for good. One evening I found myself sitting in practice with only other four other band members for company.

When I told my Mum and Dad what had been happening, they advised me to give up the band. Later Midge wrote to us, saying that she was trying to reassemble the band with a new conductor and that it would be great if I joined them. Mum said thanks, but no. I realised this was probably the best decision, although I was sad to leave the Bournemouth Silver Band and all the friends I had made there.

In the same month I watched the Munich Summer Olympics. The star of the show was a seventeen year old Russian gymnast called Olga Korbut. She stole everybody's heart, including mine. She was so pretty and talented, and she thrilled the world with her gymnastic skills, earning many gold medals in the process. I was her number one fan.

Olga Korbut is just a few years older than I am, and I still have a soft spot for her. One day I would like to take her out for dinner and thank her for spreading the appreciation of gymnastics worldwide.

Towards the end of August I organised many more

charity events, to raise money for the guide dog. I cleaned cars, and set up garage sales and mini fetes. The Guide Dogs Association gave me a large collection box topped with a moulded statue of an Alsatian. I kept the box at Ashtree House, and people sometimes put their spare change into it when they came to book riding lessons.

The total money collected from the box varied greatly from month to month – sometimes it was full to bursting, and at other times it was half empty.

One day I received a letter containing a cheque for £50. It was from an 83 year old lady, who wrote, 'Dear Antony, I hope this will help you to boost the funds for your dog'.

A week after that I had another very pleasant surprise – I was awarded a bronze medal by Mr Jones of the Guide Dogs for the Blind Association, for all my fundraising work to date. A picture was taken, of me with my medal (and Pickles the poodle!) which went into the Bournemouth Echo. Subsequently, many more donations came flooding in from local business people. Things were progressing well.

One morning, though, we were besieged by reporters from national newspapers. They had picked up on my story from the local press and wanted to follow it up. They were knocking on the windows and doors of the house, ringing the doorbell constantly, desperate to come in and talk to me and get pictures.

Mum had agreed to only speak to our local paper, the Christchurch Times, about my story, and she and Dad were annoyed by all this, and told me to hide in my room and not to look out of the window. They closed the curtains in our lounge so that the reporters could not see through into the house. One reporter was extremely persistent, shouting through the letterbox that, if we let him in, his newspaper would pay for three guide dogs!

The summer holidays were soon over, and I was back at Twynham. I found it very hard to learn because the pain was distracting me so much. I had very bad muscle spasms in my right leg. Mum noticed that my leg seemed to be getting bigger around the femur, and she took me to see Dr Cantlie again. 'Hello, Antony,' he said. 'I hear you are feeling under the weather. Let's have a look at your knee, now – try and keep straight for me while I do that, please'.

He could see that my back was bending over to the right a lot more, and he was worried about the femur, which was sticking out in different directions. 'I would like you to come back to see me again after Christmas,' he said'.

Mum asked the doctor then whether I could go back to school as usual, after Christmas. 'Yes, but if he gets any worse, you must call me immediately'.

In December, I held a mini Christmas Fayre in my Grandad's big garage at Ashtree House. There was Santa's grotto, a Tombola, a Lucky Dip, a Raffle, a bargain toy store, a sweet store, a cake store, Christmas trees for sale and refreshments. We did well, raising seventy-five pounds – but I was still five pounds short of my Guide Dog target!

Chapter Eleven
Difficult Days

The Christmas holidays flew by. Mum and Dad were worried about me though, as they could see I was struggling to get about at home. I began to use sticks to stop myself falling. My back was bending over badly, and my ribs hurt so much – I could actually hear them crunching as I walked up the stairs to my bedroom.

The worst problem was coming down the stairs, because my knee did not bend properly. I started to slide down on my bottom, but the pain from my knee was still excruciating. Mum could see that I was in a lot of distress, and made an appointment for me to see Dr Cantlie. He checked me over, looking very serious. 'Antony, it's not good news, I'm afraid,' he told me. 'I'm afraid the femur on your right leg is twice the size it was when I last saw you, and it's still growing'.

'What should we do?' asked Mum. 'Antony is due to go back to school any day now'.

'I'll write to Mr Lloyd Roberts' secretary at Great Ormond Street,' said Dr Cantlie, 'And book an appointment there for Antony. Meanwhile I'll write out a prescription for him to help with the pain from his leg and ribs. He can go back to school, but I'll ask the staff to keep a good eye on him'.

'Just get on with it,' I said to myself. 'Just do it'. The pain was very bad, but I refused to let it take over my life. I continued to work hard at school and kept taking the pain killers. My school friends were brilliant, and kept my spirits up. One of my best friends, Francis – we were like brothers – taught me to play chess. Francis and I played together, with another good friend, Ric, every lunch break – I couldn't join in with the playground games of the other children because of the discomfort, and the risk of making my health worse.

The teachers were great too – they constantly asked whether I was feeling okay, and it made me feel better to know that people were concerned and that they were watching over me.

In March I finally reached my target of £250 to buy the guide dog. At the last moment however, there was disturbing news – the target had been raised, and guide dogs now cost £500! When the local press heard, they came around to speak to me. All I could say was that I was not happy, but that I would try to reach the new target.

Two weeks later, there was good news from the Guide Dogs for the Blind Association. They said that in view of all my hard work they would break the usual rules, and let me have my dog for £250. I was delighted. And even more so when Mum arranged a big party at Ashtree House for me.

I was told that I could choose a name for the dog, and I was given a list of approved names to choose from. I was delighted to see 'Harvey' on the list. This was what I really wanted to call my dog, because Harvey was the name of the Leeds United goalkeeper and I was a Leeds fan.

In April I presented a cheque for £250 to the Guide Dogs for the Blind Association to pay for Harvey. (In fact, with the sums of money from the collection box and the various small amounts given by local businesses, I actually donated a total amount of £288.07).

My dream had come true – I had bought a Golden Labrador for a blind person! I really hoped that the dog would give that person a better life. I was going to find out who the owner was – Mr Jones had said he would contact me later in the year to let me know.

In the middle of April, my sister Julie got married. Her new husband was a sailor. Looking through the wedding pictures afterwards I was shocked – there was a photo of Julie and I with Mum and Dad, and I looked extremely unwell. I was bent over badly, and I was gritting my teeth trying to cope with the pain from my ribs and leg. I felt awful, but I was determined to put on a brave face for my sister's wedding.

It was May when I finally heard from Great Ormond Street - the letter from Mr Lloyd Roberts' secretary said that an appointment had been made for me to see the consultant on the 7th June.

Train travel was now electric, which meant that the journey was a great deal cleaner and faster. We left home at half past eight, arriving at Waterloo just two hours later. London had changed – there was no all-encompassing black smog. This time we travelled in a black taxi cab to the hospital again, but now I could see the traffic and the people much more clearly, and the air seemed so much easier to breathe.

London was fascinating and I eagerly watched it all as we passed by. There were the new skyscrapers climbing up fast as if they were in a great hurry to start new business. There were all the city people, smart and busy as if on some permanent important mission. All the noise and bustle of a huge city passing outside the taxi windows held immense excitement and satisfaction for a small boy from the country.

When I got to the hospital I got upset - I had forgotten how disturbing it was to see all those other children with their different illnesses. I was older now, and I had learned something about the miracles that were worked at Great Ormond Street – but I still couldn't help feeling scared of what was in store, both for myself and for the other children.

When we were shown in to see Mr Lloyd Roberts, he checked my knee and then sent me off for X-rays. On the way to the X-ray department, I was amazed to bump into Hanna, Jay's mother, who said Jay was in the hospital having another operation.

'Funnily enough, she was just talking about you the other day,' Hanna told me.

The X-rays were not a straightforward process. The hospital staff needed to take many X-rays, which caused me a lot of pain because I had to contort my body so that they could get close-up shots of my spine and ribs. By the time they had finished I was very tired and frightened.

Then Mum, Dad and I had to wait for the X-rays to be developed. When we went back to Mr Lloyd Roberts' office, he was flanked by medical students. They were all poring over the X-rays, and the doctor was giving instructions to his secretary. There was also another specialist present, and I struggled to understand the conversation Mr Lloyd Roberts was having with this man, in very technical-sounding medical language.

Eventually, he turned to me. 'Antony, I am very sorry to give you bad news. We need to do another operation on your right knee. The femur has grown very large, and if we don't take action it will break through your skin. Also, your back and ribs have twisted twenty degrees over to the right side. Your neck has become very stiff, and this could cause breathing problems and have a knock-on effect on your lungs. It is all very serious'.

'Will I come here to Great Ormond Street to have the operation?' I asked.

'No,' said the doctor. 'I will arrange for you to have the operation at Tadworth Court. It will be easier for your parents to visit you there. Now, Antony,' he went on. 'What we are going to do is to remove the part of the femur that is causing problems and make the right leg straighter again. After the operation you will have to lay flat on your bed for many weeks. You will have medication to ease any pain'.

'How long will Antony be in hospital for?' asked my Mum.

'It's a big operation,' said the doctor. 'I am guessing that the whole thing will take about three and a half months to heal, with perhaps another month for rehabilitation afterwards. That is, providing that everything goes smoothly'.

Mum dissolved in tears, and held onto my Dad for support. I was petrified – seeing her so upset made me realise how serious the situation was.

I had been told that I could attend school while I was waiting for the date of my operation, but I was taking a lot of pain killers, which made me feel quite weak and unwell. During the July exams I found it hard not to fall asleep, which seems hilarious in retrospect. It was not at all funny at the time though – the handwriting was making my knuckles swell and they were becoming tighter by the minute – it was like the sort of pain caused by toothache, but even worse.

It was a great relief when the exams were over, and to celebrate my friends and I went to the cinema to see the new James Bond film, Live and Let Die. It was Roger Moore's first time in the role of Bond, and it was absolutely brilliant - in fact, I can't think of a single thing about that film that I did not enjoy!

Just before the summer holidays, I received my school term and exam results. I was delighted that I had passed every subject, and the headteacher called me to his office and personally congratulated me on this achievement.

On July 27th I was admitted to hospital for an operation on my right knee (a Supraconlylar Orsteotomy). The operation took place at Tadworth Court, in ZMB ward, right next to ZMA where I had stayed back in 1969. I was introduced to the Sister, who told me that I would be given my own cubicle after the operation, so that I would have some privacy. 'You will have nice big windows to look out of,' she said, 'And the nurses will look after you well, and bring you anything you need'.

Then Mum and Dad were asked to have a chat with the Sister in her office. I was getting very nervous now. I was fourteen, considerably older than I had been at the time of my last operation, and this time I understood that I was facing a momentous challenge. When Mum and Dad came out of the Sister's office, they told me that they would be going home, but would be back the following day. 'We are going to tow our caravan to Box Hill,' Dad said, 'To keep it at a holiday camp there'.

'How long for?' I asked.

'You may be in hospital for a long while,' Dad said. 'We don't know exactly how long. But if we keep the caravan nearby it will be much easier to visit you and sleep overnight – it will cut down the number of journeys we need to make'.

Mum and Dad took me to Gatwick Airport then, to watch the planes. It was a beautiful afternoon, clear and bright, and we had tea at a cafe on a balcony which overlooked the runway. We watched the aeroplanes as they took off and landed, and had a huge fright when a Russian plane took off so close above our heads that we automatically ducked to avoid it!

When we arrived back at the hospital I began to panic, but Mum held onto me tightly. 'Listen,' she said. 'Your Dad and I have to go now, but we'll be back in the morning to see you before you go down for your operation. Is there anything you want us to bring back with us?'

Full-blown panic engulfed me then. I started to scream and shout, 'I want to go home NOW! I have had enough of hospital and I have had enough of pain! Take me home!'

Some nurses came over to calm me down. I was in a

terrible state. Dad convinced Mum that they should leave me in the care of the nurses and I calmed down once they had gone, although I was still tearful. I was in my bed now, and a nurse was holding my hand. 'It's not long now, Antony,' she said. 'You need to put a brave face on things – be strong now for your Mum and Dad. They will be with you when you go down to theatre tomorrow morning, and so will I'.

'Okay,' I said. 'I'll try'.

When I woke up in the morning there was a sign fixed to my bed, reading, 'NIL BY MOUTH'.

'What does that mean?' I asked one of the nurses.

'It means that you are not allowed anything to eat before your operation,' she replied.

I was sick from nerves anyway, and the last thing I wanted was something to eat. Then the ward sister came to see me. 'I am going to give you a 'pre-med' injection,' she said. 'It will calm you down and make you cheerful before you go into the theatre'.

I didn't feel the jab, but soon enough I was up with the birds. I started to giggle. This must be how it feels to be drunk, I thought. Two men dressed in green arrived, pushing a theatre trolley, both with blue caps covering their hair.

'Hello there,' I said cheerfully. 'Are you the tea trolley ladies, come to take me to the theatre?'

The operating theatre was next to the ward, so the hospital orderlies did not have far to push me. I was taken into a small ante-room first, and introduced to the anaesthetist. 'Hello, young man,' he said. 'I am going to put a small needle into the top of your hand now, and give you something to make you go to sleep'.

'Count to ten, please,' he continued. 'You won't get any further than eight though, before you fall fast asleep'.

I started to count to ten as I'd been instructed, but my counting was getting slower, and I'd got no further than five before I fell into a deep sleep. The operation took more than seven hours. When it was over they transferred me back to my cubicle, and laid me out on the bed, still fast asleep, flat on my back. By the time I woke up the operation was over.

It was seven o'clock in the evening. I couldn't move an inch, and all I could see was the ceiling. Eventually I managed to raise my head, and I stared down at my body. I was shocked to see myself encased in a thick plaster cast, which covered my ribs, legs and feet. I looked like a turtle.

I cried with fear, and called out for the nurses, who came running. 'What have you done to me?' I shouted. 'I can't move in this plaster. I feel numb and empty, as if a part of me is missing. What have you done to me?'

'Don't worry,' said the Sister. 'You feel like that because you still have a lot of anaesthetic in your system. It might make you feel sick too. It could take a while to work its way through, but it will eventually go. You will have to keep on being brave now. Mr Lloyd Roberts has said that you will have to be in plaster for many weeks to keep your back straight. He will be by in the morning, to have a chat with you'.

The hours crept past. At midnight a night nurse came to take my pulse and check my blood pressure. 'How are you feeling, Antony?' she asked.

'I'm having a great time,' I replied sarcastically. 'I love lying flat on my back in bed covered in plaster. I feel like a giant upside-down turtle, waiting for the tide to come in'.

The nurse smiled. 'I promise we'll look after you well, and make you as comfortable as we can,' she said.

I fell asleep then, and had some very strange dreams before I woke again at half past six the next morning. I had to struggle to remember what had happened at first, and where I was. Soon I was wide awake, and bursting for a wee.

I called out for a nurse, and she soon came, carrying a bottle. However, encased in plaster, I could not reach to use it, and so the nurse had to help me. I was a little embarrassed, but she was very kind. I was feeling very sick from the anaesthetic now, and I was told to drink plenty of water through a special straw, to clear it from my system. I was still not allowed to eat.

At about eleven o'clock Mr Lloyd Roberts appeared. 'I am pleased to tell you that the operation on your femur went very well,' he said. 'I am sorry to hear that you had a shock when you woke up and saw the plaster. How are you feeling now?'

'Not good,' I told him. 'The plaster is pressing down on my stomach and ribs and I am finding it hard to breathe'.

'Don't worry,' said the doctor. 'I know it's not a pleasant feeling, but you'll get used to that. Is there anything else you want to ask me about?'

'How will I eat?' I asked.

'You will be on a special diet that includes a lot of soft and liquid foods,' said Mr Lloyd Roberts. 'You will have a pillow behind your neck to keep your head forward, and that will make it easier for you to eat. I am afraid you may lose some weight – but I promise you won't shrink in height! You will have four pain relief injections each day, at each mealtime and at midnight, and that will help you. I have to go now, but I will see you each week to check on how you are progressing'.

Mum and Dad came to visit me then. The ward Sister was with them. 'Now, Antony,' said the Sister. 'Mr Lloyd Roberts has operated on your femur, as you know. It was twice the size of a tennis ball on your knee, so now they have broken that part, and taken all the bone away from your knee. You will have to stay on your back in bed for the next four weeks. Then you will have to go back to theatre for a plaster cast change. The new plaster will be the same shape as the old one, but a lot thicker, to keep your spine and back straight. By then your right leg should be healing, and you will feel a lot less discomfort. Your condition should be stable. Just now your body is still in shock, but soon you will be fighting a lot of pain, which is why Mr Lloyd Roberts has prescribed the painkillers. Do you understand all that?'

I said I did, and she went off and left me alone with Mum and Dad. I looked at them speechlessly. Four weeks on my back in bed! It felt like a life sentence.

Once my parents had gone back to their Box Hill caravan, a nurse brought my food in. It looked delicious - sausage chopped up into small pieces, with mashed potatoes, mashed peas and gravy.

I ate it greedily, but soon afterwards I had a messy 'accident' in my bed – it took a team of nurses more than half an hour to clean me up. 'Don't worry, Antony,' said a kind nurse. 'It's not your fault. The anaesthetic is still coming out of your system, and that is what it does to people'.

I was grateful to them for being so kind, and I soon forgot my embarrassment and laughed when the Sister said, 'That's another fine mess you got us into, Stanley!'

Just then I heard a tap on my cubicle door, and a boy came in. 'Hello there,' he said. 'My name is Nick. I had an operation on my leg last week. I went home, but I have just come back because I am having problems and I may need another operation. I am going to be here for three weeks'.

We chatted for a while, but eventually Nick had to go. 'I'll see you in the morning,' he said. 'I often help with the breakfast trolley, because the hospital are very short of nurses'.

I was very tired now, but the pain would not let me sleep. It built and built, but when I called the nurses they were all busy. Eventually Nick came back and asked whether I was okay. I told him I was not, and he promised to find a nurse and bring her back with him.

When the nurse finally arrived, she asked me to try to

relax until the Sister arrived to give me the pain-killing medication at midnight, which was only twenty minutes away. 'While we're waiting, I'll take your blood pressure,' she said.

My heart began to beat very fast. The pain was so bad that I was worried that I would faint, and the nurse was concerned because my blood pressure was so high. I panicked, and started to scream and shout out loudly. The nurse used the emergency panic button then, to call through to Tadworth Court for a duty doctor.

I was still shouting, convinced that I was going to die, and trying hard to break free of my plaster. When the doctor arrived, he gave me a pain-killing injection in my leg, and the pain vanished in seconds. My blood pressure and heart rate quickly returned to normal too.

'Don't worry, Antony,' said the doctor. 'We thought this might happen, because your body is still in shock after the operation. We will make sure that the pain is well controlled – your will have pain killers night and day if necessary. And this won't go on forever. You were in no danger this evening – you just had an adverse reaction to everything that you have been through. I promise, it will all be okay'.

The next morning, Nick arrived outside my cubicle with the breakfast trolley.
'Watch out for Matron, by the way,' he told me. 'She can be a bit of a battle-axe, and she is definitely on the warpath today. She likes to be strict, to make sure the ward runs smoothly. She reminds me of the Matron from the Carry On films'.

'I know the one,' I said. 'I'll keep an eye out for her'.

Later that morning, the pain from my leg began to creep back. I was just about to call for the nurse when the Sister turned up by my bed. 'How are you?' she asked. 'I've just come to administer your pain-killing injection'.

'I feel better already, seeing you with that needle,' I said.

While she was there she took my blood pressure and temperature, and checked my pulse rate. She kept looking at the chart, and after a while she said, 'I am just going to get a doctor to check you out'.

'Is there something wrong?' I asked.

'Your pulse is fast,' she replied, 'And you look quite red in the face. But your blood pressure seems fine. It's probably okay, but I just want to be on the safe side.'

I started to get concerned, but when the Doctor arrived to check me over, he smiled at us both. 'Antony is just suffering from this hot summer weather,' he told us. 'The thick plaster cast is causing the body heat to be trapped. He needs cooling down. I suggest we arrange for an electric fan to be fitted by the side of his bed, Sister'.

At midday, Mum and Dad arrived to visit me. The Sister told them what had happened the night before, and Mum and Dad took it well, but I could see that they were both concerned about me. At lunch time they said that they'd have to leave. 'Do you have to go so soon?' I complained. 'I am feeling very homesick'.

'I'm sorry, son,' replied my Mum. 'I have to help Grandad with the riding school. And Dad is working on a big plumbing job at a hotel in Bournemouth'.

Before they went, Nick came into the cubicle again. 'Don't worry, Mr and Mrs Evans,' he said. 'I have got a funny record to play on Antony's record player. I guarantee that it will cheer him up'.

'That's kind of you,' answered Mum. She gave me a hug then. 'Be brave,' she instructed. 'Dad and I will see you soon'.

I couldn't help being upset when my parents had gone. I knew it wouldn't be long before I saw them again – they came to see me every Wednesday and returned home the same day, and then they came back on Fridays and stayed right through the weekend. So I had company for much of the time. Despite this, though, and even though I knew I was safe and in good hands, the hospital was not an easy place to be.

From where I lay in my cubicle I could see three little boys opposite, lying in bed cots. Jamie had hip problems, and he was lying flat on his back in bed, his legs bandaged and widened out, fixed to a half moon shaped metal cradle. The second boy, Mark, had his leg in plaster. I remember one day when my Mum and Dad came to visit he called out to my Mum, 'Hello, you sexy beast!' The third boy was called Sinclair, and he also had a leg in plaster.

Mark and Sinclair were never visited by their parents, although every morning Mark would shout out to me, 'Antony, my Mum and Dad are coming to see me today!'

'Wow, that's good news Mark!' I would call back from my cubicle. But his parents never came.

Anyhow, I ate a lot for lunch that day, and afterwards I was uncomfortably full. Luckily Nick arrived then, and took my mind off it. 'You're going to be in stitches in a minute Antony,' he said, 'I've got a recording of the Goon Show for us to listen to, and it is really funny!'

'Not now, Nick,' I groaned. 'I need to rest'.

Nick seemed to be in a trance, staring at my bedside locker. Suddenly he snapped out of it. 'You have a field mouse sitting on top of your transistor radio!' he exclaimed. He somehow managed to capture the mouse, and took it cupped in his hands to the Sister's office.

Soon after that I heard several high-pitched screams, and I surmised that the nurses were terrified of the tiny mouse which Nick had innocently taken to show them! The Sister told Nick to take it away into the hospital grounds, as far as possible from the ward.

When he returned from this latest errand, he was keen to know whether my lunch had gone down yet. 'I am dying to play you the Goon Show song,' he said.

'Okay,' I answered. 'Who sings it?'

Nick told me that it was the Goon Show song, Ying Yong. It had the voices of Spike Milligan, Peter Sellers and Harry Secombe on it, and was recorded in the 1950's.

Nick was right, the record was hysterical. I was in stitches as he had predicted, and I would have been rolling on the floor if such a thing had been possible. The only problem was that it hurt to laugh – the movement made my ribs rub on the plaster. Nick told me that whenever I was homesick and feeling low he would play me the Ying Tong Song. 'It's the best cure available for homesickness,' he said.

Sometimes to alleviate the boredom of the hospital I would put my radio on, and listen to the Top 40 singles. A week after the operation I started to feel quite miserable though. I felt a lot of stress and strain from being permanently enclosed in the heavy plaster casing. One evening I decided that I would commit suicide. My plan was to shuffle across to the edge of my bed, and then push myself face down onto the ground. I was sure that this would result in my death, and I had made my mind up that this was preferable to living under such difficult conditions.

Just at the moment when I was ready to execute my plan, a nurse walked past my cubicle carrying a pile of stainless steel bedpans. Suddenly she lost control of the pans and slipped over. They made an almighty crash on the wooden floor, and jolted me out of my misery. That nurse never knew that by her comically unexpected fall she had possibly saved the life of one of her patients!

Chapter Twelve
A Home Visit

Another week passed, and I was beginning to come to terms with the situation. Mr Lloyd Roberts came to visit, and was very pleased with my progress. 'You are coping very well,' he said. 'You can go home for a week – providing your parents can arrange transport to get you there'.

'My Uncle Matt has a horse box,' I volunteered, which made him laugh.

'Good idea, Antony,' he said, 'Although not quite what I had in mind'.

The next day the ward Sister brought Mum and Dad over to my cubicle. They were all smiling. 'You're coming home with us this morning!' Mum said. I was really excited, but then a thought struck me.

'How on earth am I going to get in the Hillman Hunter with this plaster cast on?' I enquired.

'I'll show you,' said my Dad. 'I have taken the front passenger seat out of the car and made a bed. It reaches from the front dashboard to the back passenger seat'.

The nurses lifted me off my bed, helped me onto an operating theatre trolley, and wheeled me outside to the car. It felt so odd to be outside after all that time – listening to the birds sing and feeling the fresh air on my skin.

Dad opened the back side door and helped the three nurses lift me up from the trolley. I just about squeezed into the car, although it was a tight fit with my head on the back passenger seat, and my legs and feet towards the windscreen and dashboard at the front of the car.

'I've got a bottle here, in case you need a wee,' said a nurse. 'But for goodness sake don't ask for a bedpan, or your parents will have to cut the roof off the car!'

'I think Uncle Matt should have brought the horse box after all,' I said, which made the nurses start to giggle. Dad drove off then. I had a feeling I was in for a bumpy ride, and I was right. The mattress bounced up and down when we hit any irregularities in the road surface. I felt as if I was laying on a trampoline - sometimes I bumped up so high that my nose almost touched the roof of the car. It was quite an experience.

We travelled back on the motorway as slowly as possible, on the inside lane all the way. Many drivers overtook us, some of them peering into our car and looking quite surprised to see me lying flat on my back across the two seats, fully encased in plaster.

There was a heat wave that summer, and I was boiling. Mum sat next to me with a cold flannel. Before long I had to answer the call of nature and Dad looked for a lay-by in order to pull over. Then we saw a roadside sign saying, 'Next lay-by three miles' and I knew I couldn't hold on any longer. Mum got the bottle that the nurse had given us and just about managed to squeeze it in between my legs and the roof of the car, putting a pillow over the window so that no-one passing could see what was happening.

I weed into the bottle, but I had needed to go so badly that it was over-full, so that every time Mum tried to move it the urine kept spilling out. Mum told Dad that we needed to stop so that she could sort it out, and eventually we reached the lay-by, but it was so packed full with cars and coaches that we had to move on. Dad decided that the best thing would be to come off the motorway, which he did, and we quickly ended up down a country lane, and found a place to stop by the gated entrance to a field.

Thankfully Mum finally managed to move the bottle then, and I felt much more comfortable. But then I looked up, sensing a dark shadow near me by the car window. I nearly had a heart attack when the shadow came into focus – it was a mighty big bull, hanging over the gate to his field, trying to lick the car window. His face seemed bad tempered, and I imagined he was trying to tell me something, along the lines of, 'Good Mooning!'

We got back onto the motorway, and soon became stuck in a traffic jam. I felt very self-conscious as a long coach pulled up next to us, full of school-children who were all laughing at me. Dad became cross about the situation. 'If they don't start behaving themselves soon,' he said, 'I am going to get out and have a word with that coach driver'.

Luckily we arrived home without any further incident, and Dad parked the car on the driveway of our house. He looked completely shattered – I felt sorry for him. Julie came out to greet us, and she looked shocked at the sight of me. 'I have changed into a living turtle,' I said, to make her laugh.

I was carried inside, and laid on my bed, which had been moved to a corner of the lounge, facing towards the front window. It was very hard to get used to the idea of being stranded on the bed, everybody looking straight down at me.

Pickles, our poodle, came into the room then, and had a good sniff around me to find out what was going on. Even he seemed unnerved by the plaster, and not sure of what to do next. When I called his name he didn't run to me any more, but went to hide in the kitchen instead. Eventually he got used to the situation, and after that he often climbed up on top of the plaster cast to lick my face, encouraged by the fact that I couldn't move to push him off.

Mum welcomed visitors, and re-arranged the lounge furniture to accommodate them all. A lot of friends and family visited that first day, and by bedtime I was worn out. 'We're off upstairs now, Antony,' said Mum. 'Here's the broomstick. If you need anything, just use it to bang on the ceiling'.

I managed to fall asleep eventually, although I dreamed strange dreams – that I was a turtle, swimming in my plaster in the sea at Bournemouth, surrounded by hundreds of other turtles.

In the morning Ric, one of my best friends from Twynham, arrived. 'Antony,' he began, clearly embarrassed but bursting to ask me a question, 'How...how do you manage to go to the toilet? Especially if you need a poo? Do you need a crane to lift you up?'

I looked at him and laughed. I didn't answer, but just tapped my finger on the side of my nose.

My other friends from school soon arrived. It was great to see them again, and they all enjoyed signing their names on my plaster. Later that afternoon I had a big surprise – all my friends returned and our neighbours too, packing out our small house. Mum and Julie prepared a special buffet to feed them all. I was feeling a bit claustrophobic with all those people around, peering down at me, but when I told my Mum she said, 'Don't worry, Antony, it's just for a short time'.

Then I realised what all the fuss was about. Mr Jones turned up with his guide dog, and gave a speech to the assembled crowd about how I had raised money to buy a Guide Dog for the Blind. He gave me a large framed photograph of Harvey, the golden labrador I had bought and named.

It was a wonderful certificate. 'Presented to Master Antony Evans,' it said, 'In Gratitude from the Guide Dogs for the Blind Association'. I was very proud. Everyone raised three cheers, and called for me to make a speech. It felt odd, lying on my back speaking to the ceiling, but I did my best.

'Thank you everyone for coming here today,' I announced. 'I am delighted that I managed to buy Harvey. It all began when I was at Great Ormond Street Hospital in 1967. So many people bought me sweets to cheer me up after my operation that I decided I could either eat them all and get fat, or sell them to help other people. So I sold them, and decided to use the money to benefit the blind – and to cut a long story short, after a long period of fund-raising, in April this year I finally raised enough money to buy a guide dog for the blind. I am really pleased to have been able to help in this way'.

When I finished my speech I was rewarded with a loud cheer, and then everyone burst out singing, 'For he's a jolly good fellow!' At that point a reporter and photographer from our local paper came into the lounge. Mr Jones spoke to the reporter, and told him that I was the only disabled child in the whole of the United Kingdom who had bought a guide dog for the blind.

Later that same day there was an article on the front page of the paper about me – it was a wonderful story – and a picture to go with it. I felt a bit shocked when I saw myself in that photo, looking pale and tired, like a ghost covered in a plaster cast.

In the evening the phone rang off the hook – there were hundreds of people living around Christchurch and Bournemouth who wanted to congratulate me after reading the article in the paper. Mum told me that one of the callers was the Mayor of Christchurch, Mr Staniforth, and that he would be coming to see me the next morning with my headteacher, Mr Cotton.

When I woke up the next day, I was in a lot of pain – my right knee was hurting at the site of the operation. I was in agony, so Mum gave me two painkillers, tablets which would also help me to relax and stay calm. They caused another problem though – I found it hard to speak and started to feel a bit wobbly and giggly, as though I'd had too much to drink.

Mum laughed and told me not to worry about it, 'It's only the tablets making you feel a bit funny, Antony,' she said.

When the two men arrived, the Mayor was very kind. He said that he had put me on his prize giving award list because of my bravery. 'And,' he went on, 'Mr Cotton here has told me all about how hard you work at school'.

Julie spoke to Mr Cotton, while the Mayor signed his name on my plaster. 'I hope you get well soon,' he told me. 'Don't worry if you can't make it to the prize-giving – I'll sort something special out'.

Mr Cotton spoke then. 'In September, when the school term starts, Antony, I will mention you, and we'll all say a short prayer for you'.

Mum was overcome by the kindness of Mr Cotton and the Mayor. 'I am going to get through this whatever happens,' I said to them. 'I know it is going to be very tough for me. This is only the beginning. But I know I will find a way through'.

It was time for the Mayor to leave then. Before he went we had a quick word. 'When you come home again Antony,' he said, 'Hopefully in about two weeks' time, I will arrange for your prize award to be presented to you. Keep focusing on getting better now. Bye!' And off he rode on his bicycle back to the town hall in Christchurch.

Mr Cotton stayed a while longer, chatting with my Mum and Dad. 'When Antony comes home,' he told them, 'I will arrange for him to have free home tuition until he is well enough to return to school'.

My Mum and Dad were really grateful. 'We don't know when Antony will be able to return to school,' said my Dad, 'Because after the plaster is off he will need to learn to walk all over again. It could be January or February next year before he is able to go back to school'.

'It doesn't matter how long it takes,' said my headteacher, 'Antony is a very well known and respected member of the school and we will always be pleased to welcome him back. He will know when he is ready to return to Twynham. Meanwhile, we'll keep him on track with his school work, don't worry about that'.

The next day, Uncle Matt arrived with a surprise. He had arranged for a special metal framed bed to be made for me with wheels attached. Matt knew how much I liked going to see the Regatta fireworks display, and was determined that I would not miss out this year.

I eyed the contraption warily. 'I hope you haven't nicked this from an ambulance,' I said.

Matt laughed. 'Who do you think I am?' he said. 'I wouldn't do that. Or would I? Actually,' he went on, 'I got your Dad to measure you when you were asleep, so that I could give a plan drawing to Priory Engineering, who built the bed for me'.

'It's really kind of you,' I said to my Uncle. 'But how is this going to work?'

'Just you wait and see,' said Matt.

Some of the Ashtree Riding School staff came over to help my Dad lift me into his car, and we set off to Hengistbury Head. Just as we arrived Uncle Matt turned up, with the Landrover and box trailer. He parked in the golf club car park, opened the box trailer and wheeled out the bed. It was like something out of Thunderbird 4!

Matt ignored the crowd of bystanders who had gathered to gawp at the spectacle, and wheeled the bed over to my Dad's car. It was only when the bystanders failed to disperse that we realised these people were not just interested to see what was going to happen next with the bed. Because of the horse box, they thought there was going to be a chance of pony rides. Matt had to set everybody straight on that one, and they eventually wandered off.

I was moved by the riding school staff again then, from Dad's car to the metal framed bed. Mum covered me with blankets, and Uncle Matt told me to hold tight, because we were ready to roll. 'We're going to wheel you down a stony footpath now,' he said. 'It might be a bit bumpy'.

Well, bumpy was an understatement. I felt as though I was riding along that footpath in a wagon train from a Western movie, vibrating up and down all the way. I was terrified that I would come a cropper. I also had an audience to contend with – hundreds of people all looking down at me open-mouthed, wondering what on earth I was doing there.

The fireworks started just as we got to the river. It was a brilliant display, but marred by groups of children who were pointing at me and laughing. Matters got worse when a dog approached, and still attached to the lead held by his owner, weed onto my plaster to mark what he considered to be his territory. To add injury to insult, the disgusting mutt then started licking my face enthusiastically. It was a revolting and embarrassing experience.

I was so pleased when we finally arrived home. I did

not want Matt to think that I was ungrateful though, and I thanked him for going to such a lot of trouble and expense, getting a special mobile bed made just so that I could see the fireworks.

Chapter Thirteen
Ups and Downs

It was soon time to return to Tadworth Court. My week at home seemed to have passed very quickly. Nanny and Grandad came over to pay a quick visit before I left. As Dad and our next door neighbour picked me up, Julie picked up Pickles the poodle, and both of them waved goodbye to me (although I think Julie might have been moving Pickles' paw!)

The weather was still hot, although the temperature had dropped a little since the heatwave of the previous week. We arrived at Tadworth Court without incident, and I settled down, and asked a passing nurse for news of Nick. 'I'm afraid he has gone back home,' she said. 'He couldn't have his operation after all. He left a message for you though. He asked me to tell you not to give up, and to keep playing the Ying Tong song'. She pointed over to my locker, and I saw that Nick had left me the vinyl single of the Ying Tong song, by the Goons.

I was sad not to have had the chance to say goodbye to Nick. I was very pleased to have met him though – he had encouraged me to have hope, and to concentrate on getting well. Jamie was not in his bed either, and the nurses said that he had been transferred back to the Great Ormond Street hospital. Sinclair and Mark were still in their cots. I asked the nurse whether they'd had any visitors in the week since I had left, and she looked sad and said that no, they had not. The good news was that they were now allowed to be pushed out into the grounds in their wheelchairs – so there was progress.

The next day I had to go to the operating theatre to have my plaster changed. My body temperature had caused it to start to crack and shatter, and there was an awful smell emanating from it. I had to be put under a general anaesthetic for three or four hours while the plaster was changed and I woke up feeling very odd. The new plaster cast was the same shape but a lot thicker, and it felt tighter around my body and legs.

The sister came to my bedside to check my pulse. 'Did you have any good dreams while you were in theatre?' she asked.

'I don't remember,' I told her. 'Why?'

'You kept calling for Pickles,' she replied. 'Whoever is Pickles?'

'He's my pet poodle,' I answered. 'Did I say anything else?'

'You told Pickles off for weeing on your plaster,' she laughed.

'He's never done that!' I exclaimed. 'I must have dreamt it because of what happened when I was at home. My uncle took me to watch the fireworks in a special bed, and a dog cocked his leg and did a wee over the side of my plaster'.

'No wonder it smelled,' laughed the Sister. 'Did that really happen?'

I assured her that it had, and she went red in the face from laughing, and begged for more details of the incident. I told her that I was saying no more, because it was far too embarrassing. I was glad to have made her laugh though.

Later in the day, Mum and Dad came over to see me – they were staying in the caravan at Box Hill. I was still very tired from the anaesthetic, and was struggling to keep my eyes open. The Sister spoke to us all. 'You are going to have to stay here for a week and a half now, Antony, because the plaster needs to dry out,' she said. 'I want your Mum and Dad to have a break back at home. Do you understand what I am saying?'

'Of course I do, Sister,' I said. 'That's fine by me'.

Mum and Dad both gave me a huge hug, looking very relieved. 'I was worried you might be upset,' confided Mum. 'Thank you for being so good about it all. It is a big help to us'.

'Don't worry about me,' I told them. 'I have got all the nurses to look after me, and I am quite used to being in plaster now'.

'Is it okay if we go home today?' asked Mum nervously.

'You'd better go right now, before I change my mind!' I joked.

A week passed since the plaster change, and I started to get very fed up. The new cast chafed on my lower spine. I told the Sister in charge, and she brought a doctor, who rolled me over onto my side and used a small torch to look inside the plaster.

'I have slid some cotton wool inside the plaster,' he told me afterwards. 'That should do the trick'. I felt a lot better now, and I was glad that I had asked for help. Soon after that, Mum and Dad came to collect me and take me home again. By the time we got there, the plaster cast had started to rub again, and began to feel quite painful. I was pleased to be home, but very tired and desperate for a good sleep.

The next morning the postman arrived. He had brought two parcels, which he handed over to Mum and Julie. They came into the lounge with Dad, all smiling at me. 'Julie has something to tell you, Antony,' said Mum.

Julie handed me a letter. When I opened the envelope I could hardly believe my eyes. I went into a cold sweat in that hot plaster cast. I was looking at a letter addressed to me, from the Leeds United Football Club manager Don Revie! And with it was a photograph of the team and a page of autographs signed by all of them! Even David Harvey, my all-time favourite goalkeeper (who I had named Harvey the Guide Dog after) was there.

It was an astonishing surprise. And there was more to come – another parcel, this one in the shape of a long tube. I opened the lid and slid the contents out. It was a rolled up sheet of paper tied with a red ribbon. Mum helped me to open it out and she shouted out with joy, 'Oh that's fantastic!'

It was the prize-giving award from Mr Staniforth, the Mayor. I had been awarded a certificate from Christchurch Borough Council, embossed with the special council crest which bore the words, 'For Fidelity and Freedom'. The mayor had written on it, 'To Antony with best wishes, Tom Staniforth, Mayor of Christchurch,' and the date, 13th September 1973. I felt so honoured, and I really appreciated the Mayor taking the trouble to do this for me.

I was so happy, and yet I was still in pain. I was having a difficult time with my plaster and as the day wore on I began to get quite edgy. I hated to complain, but the plaster kept rubbing on my spine, and it got so bad that I felt as though I was being stabbed with a sharp stake.

Mum and Dad tried to look into my plaster to see the source of the pain. They noticed that there was a lot of blood spilling out of my back. Mum panicked then, and immediately rang the hospital. The sister said that I must be brought back as soon as possible.

Our neighbour arrived at 6am the following day, to help Dad get me into the car. Every time I moved, the plaster dug into my spine, sending excruciating jolts through my entire body. Mum managed to keep me on my side, with a cushion behind me to ease the pressure, but the pain was razor sharp, and it made the journey extremely unpleasant.

It was 10am before we reached Ward ZMB. The nurses wheeled me over to the treatment room immediately, on an operating trolley as usual. A doctor moved me gently onto my side, and used a special metal cutting tool to cut a 'V' shape out of the plaster. He and the nurse were clearly very disturbed by what they saw.

'How on earth did that happen?' said the Doctor. 'Oh blimey!' (He actually used stronger language than that!) 'Antony,' he said to me, 'I am really sorry that this has happened to you. I can see exactly why you have been so uncomfortable – the plaster rubbing on you has ended up cutting through your skin. We'll dress the wound for you now, and then you can go back home'.

My poor father was still very tired from the journey up to Tadworth Court. 'Okay, come on Antony,' he said. 'Let's get cracking, before I start nodding off again'. And so we set off once more, on the long trip back to Christchurch. When we reached home, Dad asked Mum to ring Grandad and Uncle Matt, to ask if they could come to help him lift me out of the car. When they arrived, though, Grandad said that he didn't need any help, he could lift me himself.

True to his word, he picked me up and carried me from the car into the house, laying me onto my bed in the lounge, as if I weighed no more than a feather. 'How did you manage to do that, Grandad?' I asked.

'I have been in the fruit and vegetable business a long time,' he replied. 'I may be an old man, but I can still carry a sack of potatoes'.

'Yes, but I am not a sack of potatoes!' I protested.

During the next few days at home I received literally stacks of parcels, letters and get well cards. Julie read out all the cards to me, and I enjoyed listening to her. She sounded very professional, as if she was on 'Jackanory,' a popular BBC programme of that time.

I was a bit lonely at times during the day, because all my friends had gone back to school. I found various ways to keep myself amused when I was alone, listening to the radio or browsing through my 'Look-In' magazines – I had a full collection of these. 'Look-In' was a minefield of information and entertainment.

I always listened to Terry Wogan on Radio Two, early in

the morning.   Later in the morning, Jimmy Young would come on, in 'The JY Prog'. I liked him, with his various catchphrases - and of course, he played some great music.

In the afternoons I listened to 'Diddy' David Hamilton's afternoon show – he played some of the top ten hits, and asked music questions for callers to answer. And in the evening I watched television.   That way, the time passed, each day much like the one before.

On my last day at home, the whole family played all sorts of games together in the lounge. I was staring out of the window, watching my friends outside playing on their bikes or kicking balls about.   I started to cry. 'What's the matter, son?' asked my Mum. 'Are you in a lot of pain?'

'It's not that,' I said. 'I just wish I was outside with my friends'.

'You soon will be,' my Mum replied. 'It won't be long now'. Pickles stayed extra close to me all through that day, as if he was trying to cuddle into my plaster. I'm sure he must have known that I was going back to hospital the next day – he looked so sad.

It was now the end of the first week in September. Early in the morning we set off to Tadworth Court once more, for my final stay in Ward ZMB.   Dad was getting stressed out with all the pressure and the long journeys to and from the hospital. He said that he hoped this would be the last time he would have to convert his car to accommodate me, my plaster and my mattress.   If things went according to plan, on the way home next time, I should be able to sit up as usual!

All three of us were in a bad frame of mind that morning though. Mum was finding things difficult – everything seemed to be getting on top of her. She was juggling a lot of balls – she was busy trying to help Grandad with the riding business at Ashtree House, as well as dealing with my trips to and from the hospital, and managing the household.

Dad had to cope with the worry of trying to keep his plumbing business afloat, and had to keep cancelling jobs because of my hospital stays. And I was upset, in pain as usual and bad tempered, fed up from lying down on my back with nothing to look at but the ceiling every day.

I slept soundly that night in hospital, but somehow it seemed as though only five minutes had passed when I woke up again. My eyes were full of sleepy dust and there was no way to shift it with my body encased in plaster. I was uncomfortable – I had lost weight, and so although the cast had been designed to fit firmly around my body, I felt as though I was rattling around loose inside it. I simply could not wait for all this to be over.

In the middle of the morning Mum and Dad came to visit me. 'There is a garden fete in the grounds outside,' a nurse told them. 'I suppose you want to go, do you, Antony?' All three of us smiled in anticipation. 'I'll have to think about how to get you out there,' said the Nurse. 'Hang on a minute'.

She disappeared off, and Mum and Dad and I waited to see if she would come up with some method to get me outside. Meanwhile, we could see all the other children being taken out – some in wheelchairs, some in wheeled chariots, and some in bath tubs on wheels.

Before long, the nurse re-appeared. There was another nurse with her, and they were pushing an operating trolley with an oxygen bottle still fixed to it. 'Here's your taxi, Sir,' announced the nurses, laughing at our surprise. Between them, the nurses lifted me onto the trolley, and Mum and Dad pushed me outside, through the long path with the archway above, towards the main gardens where the fete was being held.

There were all sorts of activities taking place. Nurses were running in an egg and spoon race. Mums and Dads were running in a pancake race. There was a fancy dress competition, a hook-a-duck stall and a coconut shy. There was a candy floss stall, a plant stall, an ice cream parlour...

Dad saw me looking at the ice cream parlour. 'Would you like an ice-cream?' he asked. 'Oh yes please!' I exclaimed. He went off, and came back with a '99', a whippy vanilla ice cream with a chocolate flake. Mum held it, and I attacked it greedily. But the sun was warm that day and the ice-cream melted faster than I could get to it. It is hard eating an ice-cream when somebody else is holding it for you, and before long I was in a sticky mess, plaster covered in ice-cream, face covered in ice cream... I didn't mind though, it tasted delicious.

One of the doctors was running the Hoopla stall, calling out like he was at a fairground, 'Roll up, roll up, try your luck at the Hoopla!' I couldn't take part in any of it, of course, but I was just happy to be there, watching everybody else enjoying themselves.

'Why are you holding a summer fete in September?' Dad

asked a passing nurse.

'We have a fete every year. It was supposed to be last week,' she replied. 'But we had very bad thunderstorms so we changed the date. I'm glad Antony didn't miss out – he came back just in time to join us for the fun today'.

'The brass band are trying hard,' said my mother diplomatically. 'Antony used to play with the Bournemouth Silver Band. He played a beautiful Austrian cornet'.

'Hold on a minute,' said the nurse. 'I'll be back soon. Keep eating that ice-cream, Antony – or should I say, wearing it!' She reappeared seconds later with the conductor of the band. He held a silver cornet.

'I hear you used to play,' he said. 'Would you like to have a go on this?'

'I would, please,' I said. 'But I might be a little rusty'. I tried to blow into the cornet, but I couldn't make a sound. It was hopeless – I just could not muster the energy that the instrument required. I felt a bit embarrassed, but the conductor told me not to worry.

'At least you had a go,' he said.

I enjoyed my time at the garden fete very much. It was wonderful to see everybody enjoying themselves, and I was sad when it was time to return to the ward. 'You're going to be having X-rays tomorrow,' said my Mum, 'To see whether your knee has healed yet. If it hasn't, apparently you could be in plaster for a little longer than was planned. Sorry to have to tell you that. The Sister says you can call us tomorrow night at 7pm to tell us what the decision is'.

They went off to their caravan, and later that evening a nurse came by to see me. 'What's up, Antony?' she asked. 'I can tell that there's something bothering you'.

'There's something scary about my body,' I said.

'Oh dear, have you turned into a ghost?' she quipped.

'No, it's worse than that,' I told her. 'If I look down the top half of my plaster cast I can see my ribs sticking out, and my body has completely shrunk. If I move my legs in the plaster they feel like matchsticks'.

'Hold on a minute,' said the nurse. 'I'll ask Sister to come and have a look at you'.

The Sister arrived and examined me closely. She said, 'You certainly have lost a lot of weight Antony. Your stomach is about an inch away from the plaster and your ribs are protruding'.

'Is it serious?' I asked.

'Well, Mr Lloyd Roberts did say it might happen,' replied the Sister. 'Don't let's worry about it now – tomorrow we'll get the results from your X-rays and we'll know more'.

I couldn't get to sleep that night. I lay on my back counting imaginary sheep, but that didn't help. So instead I counted horses taking the jumps at Ashtree Riding School which did the trick – before I knew it a nurse had come to wake me.

'Hurry up and get out of bed, Antony!' said the nurse. 'Quick as you can please – we need to change the sheets'.

'Hang on a minute!' I said. 'I'm covered in plaster and I'm not going anywhere in a hurry, thank you very much'.

'Gotcha!' said the nurse, giggling.

After the X-rays were done, one of the nurses stopped to speak to me. 'I've seen your X-rays,' she said, 'And the bones on your knee have joined together well. Your back and ribs are a lot straighter'. I was really happy to hear this, but knew that I shouldn't relax - I would have to wait to hear the official verdict from the specialist.

When I got back to the ward a lady was waiting outside my cubicle. She asked whether I would like to take part in a cookery lesson with some of the other children. They were making shortbread. 'Ooh, yes please!' I replied. 'But how am I going to do that, lying flat on my back in bed?'

'It'll be fine,' she said. 'We'll lay a mixing bowl on top of your plaster. One of the nurses can supervise you'.

The nurse put a cloth on top of my plaster, and laid the mixing bowl on top of it (this was to stop the bowl slipping off). Then she put butter into the bowl, and I started to beat it until it went creamy. Next she poured in caster sugar, which I had to stir around with a wooden spoon. Then I had to sieve some plain flour into the bowl. The nurse and I couldn't help laughing at this point – there was more flour on me than there was in the bowl.

The nurse then held the bowl fast, and tilted it so that I could mix and blend the creamy butter, sugar and flour together. It went into a thick dough, and I used my hands to shape it. Now I had to use a rolling pin to roll the thick dough until it was only 3mm deep. The nurse put a wooden pastry board on top of my plaster so that I could do this. But I was struggling to get my head down to see what I was doing.

'Hang on a minute,' said the nurse. 'I'll go to the store room and see if I can find a mirror'.

She came back with a small mirror, which she held above my head so that I could see myself rolling out the dough. 'Hurry up, Antony,' she soon said. 'My arms are killing me!'

'Don't worry,' I said, 'I've nearly finished now. Just another half an hour'.

'If you weren't in plaster,' she said, 'I'd empty that bag of flour over your head!'

We both laughed. The cookery teacher came back at that point, tapped on the window of the cubicle and came in. 'It looks as though you two have had a great time,' she said.

'It reminds me of the time I made a model of Stonehenge out of clay, at school,' I said. 'Maybe I could make one out of shortbread'.

'Hmm,' responded the cookery teacher. 'That sounds like a very interesting idea. We'll have to try that one day'. The teacher told the nurse to cut the dough into ten finger strips and put them on a baking tray. Then she took these off to be baked in the oven. It had been so much fun making shortbread – now all I had to do was wait for it to be cooked.

At 4pm the nurse brought the afternoon tea trolley, which was always stocked with delicious home-made cakes. 'I have something for you,' said the nurse. 'I think you should be very proud of what you have achieved today, Antony'.

She passed me a small white bag, and inside I found my shortbread finger sticks. They looked brilliant, and when I bit into one I found that they tasted pretty good too. I was pleased to be able to give one to the nurse who had helped me make them, and I couldn't wait to be able to give one to my Mum and Dad when they came to visit.

A nurse came in to check on me after the evening meal. 'I'll be back with your painkillers as soon as Coronation Street has finished,' she called over her shoulder as she sped back to the playroom.

'What a cheek!' I called back, 'Leaving me like this just so you can go and watch TV!'

I didn't mean it of course – the nurses were the best thing about being in hospital. They worked hard on the wards, doing a marvellous job for us all, but they always had time for a bit of fun and laughter – which was medicinal in itself!

The next day was very warm again. A nurse asked whether I would like to be wheeled outside in my bed, and I eagerly agreed. The bed was wheeled onto the veranda, which was amazing. There were lots of children out there, some of us in our beds, and some scooting around in their wheelchairs or wheeled chariots.

Those of us in bed played games with the nurses. I played Happy Families, and was on a lucky streak – I won almost every game. 'How on earth do you manage to keep on winning, Antony?' said the nurse eventually. 'It feels so unfair! I think you should play the champion now – she's standing right behind you'.

'Who's the champion?' I asked, because of course I couldn't turn around to look. But then I heard a voice, 'Hello, little brother!'

It was my sister Julie. I felt numb with the shock. Julie hugged me, and I cried with joy to see her – I had missed her a lot. Mum and Dad were there too – I had not expected to see any of them that day, and it was a wonderful surprise. I almost felt I was dreaming – but the three of them soon assured me that they were not a figment of my imagination!

Julie said that she was really pleased to get the opportunity to see Tadworth Court at last, so I asked a nurse whether she would mind wheeling me back inside so that I could show Julie my cubicle. Our parents came too, and Mum noticed the bag of shortbread on top of my locker.

'Where did you get the shortbread from, Antony?' she asked.

'I made it yesterday,' I said, and my Mum began to laugh.

'Oh, pull the other one,' she said. 'How could you have been making shortbread when you are stuck on your back in bed?'

Just at that moment, a nurse popped her head in around the door. 'He did make the shortbread and I helped him,' she said, and everybody laughed. Dad licked his lips hungrily. 'I am a bit peckish, as it happens,' he said. 'Could I have a taste, please?'

Julie had her slice first. She took a bite, then gave me an odd look. 'There's too much salt in this,' she said.

'I didn't add any salt to it' I told her.

'I was just being silly,' she laughed. 'It's delicious really. Well done Antony'.

Between them, my family ate up all the shortbread. 'That's one pound and fifty pence please,' I said, after I had watched them finish it all off, and I held out my hand. 'It's nice to do business with you!'

'What a cheek you have!' my Mum exclaimed. Then Mum and Dad went off to have another chat with the Ward Sister in her office.

Julie and I were alone now, and she looked at me seriously. 'How are you coping with all this, Antony?' she asked.

'I don't know,' I said. 'I feel very weak. I've lost weight. And sometimes I think I can't cope with being in this plaster for a minute longer. I get panicky and then I can't help thinking I am going to die. And if I don't die,

I am afraid that I will look like a skeleton anyway, when I come out of the plaster. And apart from all that, I'm worried about Dad. He doesn't look at all well'.

Julie just held my hand tight to comfort me, and that is how Mum and Dad found us when they came back into the cubicle. They were both smiling. 'The Sister has good news for you, Antony,' Mum said.

The Sister came in then, followed by an Indian doctor. 'Hello, Antony,' he said. 'Mr Lloyd Roberts asked me to check your x-rays, and I have had a good look at them. Everything has turned out very well. I am pleased to say that your knee has completely healed now, and your back and ribs are a great deal straighter than before. Tomorrow morning you will come out of your plaster for good. There are some things you need to know about the procedure'.

'We will be using a small round electric cutting blade,' he went on, 'To cut out each side of your plaster cast. This will be very noisy. Then we will remove the top half of the cast, and after that, the bottom half. When you first come out of the plaster, your body will smell very bad. There will also be steam coming off your body. All this is normal, but it may make you feel sick'.

I was feeling sick already, but I asked the doctor to continue. 'I want you to be aware of how you will look,' he said, 'Your back will be very straight. But your body will have shrunk because you have lost weight. Your stomach will be flat like a pancake, the bones from your legs and rib cage will be protruding. Even your skin will look different – because you have had the plaster on for so long your skin will look brown and will feel itchy. It will start to flake off over the next few days. All these things are normal when somebody has been in a full body plaster, and it will not take long before your body returns to its usual condition. But I want you to be aware of these things, so that you are not shocked by them'.

The doctor had explained everything very thoroughly, which I appreciated, and I thanked him but I still felt nervous. Mum and Dad recognised that I was edgy in the face of this next challenge. Mum said that this was great progress though, just what we had all been hoping for. 'By tomorrow afternoon you'll be running around the ward and jumping for joy,' she smiled.

They all left then, and I was alone again. I lay on my back, gazing at the ceiling, feeling quite helpless. I was so confused – I felt like shouting, screaming or crying, and I didn't know where all these emotions had come from. We had all battled for so long, and now it seemed that the struggle might be over at last. No more plaster ever again – how great that would be!

The next morning after I awoke, I was wheeled down to the treatment room at the end of the ward. I was lifted off my bed, and laid down onto a plastic mattress.

'Don't be scared, Antony,' said the Sister. 'We have done this hundreds of times before. I promise that the machine we use to cut the plaster off will not hurt you at all. Take deep breaths now, and that will help to keep you calm'.

Then I heard what sounded like the vibrations of a small chainsaw, as my plaster was slowly cut in two. Several nurses held me tight, so that I could not move. A thick white dust came up, which felt like talcum powder and created a cloud so dense that I could not see at all. I wondered how the nurses could possibly know what they were doing.

Finally they finished cutting around the plaster, and gently lifted the top half of the cast off my body. It was quite a job, as it seemed to be stuck in place with thick green stringy padding. I managed to tilt my head forward, and saw the top half of my body for the first time in months.

The doctor had been right – there was an awful smell, so overpowering that I felt faint, and I was given oxygen to help me breathe. I felt as though I was in a horror film.

Now it was time to take the bottom half of the cast off – but that was stuck to me even more firmly. I looked and felt like a jelly waiting to be pulled out of its mould, and meanwhile the air felt very strange on the top of my body. It was surreal.

The nurses tugged and tugged, but the plaster wouldn't budge, and eventually they had to call for reinforcements. With the help of the extra staff, the plaster finally came off. Instead of a turtle, I now looked like a newborn chick, just hatched from a shell.

My legs looked like burnt matchsticks, and I could not stop them from shaking. My temperature kept changing from hot to cold and back again. The right leg, where the overgrown femur had made my knee the size of two tennis balls, had now returned to a normal appearance and looked completely healed, again just as the Indian doctor had forecast.

The nurses wrapped me up to keep me comfortable, and

moved me back over to my bed. They said that I would have to stay there, still flat on my back, for the next twenty-four hours. The same doctor came back to see me then. 'I bet that is a relief, Antony, getting that plaster off you,' he said. 'You have done so well – I am really pleased. How do you feel?'

'Like a newborn chicken,' I said, which made him smile. ' I also have the strangest feeling – as though I am about to float up to the ceiling'.

'That is to be expected,' the doctor replied. 'You have just had the weight off the plaster taken off you, so it is usual that you would feel some strange sensations. But what I would like to know is whether you are in any pain at all'.

I looked at him then, and it dawned upon me that for the first time for as long as I could remember I was actually feeling no pain at all. 'The truth is, Doctor,' I told him, 'The pain has completely gone!'

'That is just what we had hoped for,' he replied. 'I do have to put a plaster splint under your right leg now though, to keep it straight. Your knee is still locked, and so after a day in bed you will start a programme of physiotherapy to unlock and bend it. Meanwhile, you will also be getting accustomed to sitting up in bed – you have been lying horizontally for so long that it will feel very disorientating to become vertical again. You will also be given plenty of bed baths, for obvious reasons'.

I did feel strange, lying flat on my back in the bed. My body felt unstable without the weight of the plaster to tether it, and so although I knew I was on earth, I felt somehow as if I was floating in space. I felt as though my body was drifting away from the bed, leaving just my soul behind. It was very strange. I began to imagine that I was a skeleton, riding in a ghost train...

Luckily I had the nursing staff to take care of me. I was wearing a long white hospital gown at that point. One of the nurses said that she was going to warm me up – but, she told me, 'I will have to put this half-circle metal frame over your bed, and drape the blanket over that, so that the bed covers don't rub on your skin and on the scar from your operation'.

Once she had done that I felt warmer and more comfortable, but then I looked down at myself and started to laugh. 'What's so funny?' the nurse asked, mystified.

'I look like a pregnant lady about to give birth to twins!' I exclaimed, and she burst out laughing too. Eventually she managed to control herself and went off to see the other children on her round. But every hour after that, one or other of the nurses would pop their head around the door of my cubicle to ask whether my twins had arrived yet. 'No!' I would call back. 'Go away, you silly lot!'

I ate a lot that day – the staff must have been concerned at my weight loss because they set about feeding me up immediately. I was given many cups of tea, heavily sugared, which I still drank with my special straw. And supper time was especially enjoyable - I could finally eat more solid food, which was great.

For the first three days after my plaster came off, I had special physiotherapy treatment, to learn to bend my knee again (the splint applied by the Indian doctor had been taken off by now). I asked the physiotherapist about my stitches, and she told me that they were dissolving ones which had already disappeared without any trace. I was pleased not to have to go through any more procedures.

The physiotherapy was painful, although I was glad to have the chance to improve my mobility. It gave me something to focus on, and each day I made good progress. By the end of the week I was delighted that I could bend my knee again. The next plan, the physiotherapist told me, was to learn to sit up on my bed – I was still lying flat on my back at that point, to stop the room spinning.

The evening of the day that I learned to bend my knee, a nurse knocked on the door of my cubicle. 'How would you like to phone your Mum and Dad tonight?' she asked, 'And give them the good news?'

'That would be great, nurse,' I replied. 'But how will I get to the telephone?'

'We'll bring it to you,' she replied. 'We have a long extendable wire on the telephone, and I'm sure we can reach your cubicle'.

So I called my Mum and Dad, still lying flat on my back in bed. I am not sure how I managed to dial the numbers on the telephone, but I did. Mum was really pleased to speak to me, and after a while she said, 'Hang on a minute. There's somebody else here who wants to talk to you'.

I was confused for a minute, as all I could hear was a

series of heavy snuffling and sniffing noises. Then the penny dropped. It was my pet poodle on the phone. 'It's you, Pickles!' I burst out. Then Mum began chatting away again. 'Is that still you talking, Pickles?' I asked.

'No, it's your mother!' she replied, and I could not stop laughing. Eventually I told Mum the good news, that I could bend my knee again. I explained to her that I was feeling a lot better, but not looking forward to having to sit up on my bed the next day. I was frightened in case the room began spinning again.

'You'll be fine, Antony,' my Mum reassured me. 'The worst of it is over now. We'll come to see you soon. Bye, son!'

Next morning I woke up early. The physiotherapist soon came into my room. 'Right, Antony,' she said. 'You know what the plan is. We are going to sit you up straight on your bed very slowly. We will hold on tightly to you, so that you don't fall over'.

'Okay...' I replied hesitantly.

'Once we have you straight, you might feel very giddy and sick, but don't panic. This is just the effect of the blood's circulation getting in order again, running away from your head and down your legs. You have been flat on your back in bed for a very long time, and your body has got to get used to everything again'.

'How long will it take for my body to get used to being up straight?' I asked.

'You'll be back to normal again in two or three days,' she replied. 'You will have to sleep sitting up for a while, using a back rest fixed to the bed. This will help you to recover faster'.

The physiotherapist and her assistant gently pulled me up to sitting. This felt really peculiar – the cubicle and the whole ward it was in span around fast, as if I was a piece of clothing in a washing machine. I began to panic.

My legs felt completely numb, which was unnerving. Then I felt hot and cold alternately, all over my body. The nausea took hold, and I couldn't control it – I was sick all over the floor. I panicked - shouting, screaming and crying uncontrollably.

The physiotherapists had to call extra nursing staff to hold me down. I was convinced that I was going to die, and I could already feel myself drifting away from everybody. Eventually the nurses managed to calm me, although I was still very shaky. Then they decided to fix a cradle rest to my bed, to keep me in an upright position.

The Indian doctor was called to check on me. 'I hear you had a problem sitting up,' he said.

'It was terrible,' I told him. 'I thought I was going to die'.

'You are not going to die now,' said the doctor cheerfully. 'In just a few days you will be smiling again. The good news is that everything is going well, but just as we expected it will take you a little while to adjust to being upright again'.

Before he left, the doctor checked my blood pressure and looked into my eyes, to make sure that I was well.

He also asked if I had any pain. Luckily I had no pain at all, and I also felt a lot calmer and more confident after seeing the Indian doctor. I knew that I just had to work hard now on my back exercises, and set my sights on learning to walk again – my next challenge!

During the next week I started to feel much happier. I worked hard with the physiotherapist, and everything was going smoothly. One morning I heard a tap on my cubicle door. 'Come in!' I called.

A large lady wearing a white plastic apron stood in my room. 'It's time for your bed bath, Antony,' she said.

'Not now,' I said. 'Please'.

She laughed merrily. 'Where shall I start?' she asked.

'Don't touch my arms,' I said. 'I have had lots of injections and they are badly bruised and they hurt'.

'I won't hurt anybody,' the nurse said. 'I am completely harmless'. She then took an enormous scrubbing brush from her bag, harsh and wiry, something that would usually be used to clean floors. 'I am going to use this brush to get all the flaky skin off your back,' she announced. I was very alarmed, and could feel my face turning quite red.

She laughed again, an outrageously loud and infectious laugh, and at the same time she shouted out, 'Gotcha! You should have seen your little face! Let me introduce myself properly, Antony,' she went on. 'My name is Winnie. I am going to be doing your bed baths twice a day, to clean you up. Apparently you have been stinking the whole ward out'.

'Thank goodness you were joking about that scrubbing brush!' I said. 'I thought you had come from another planet'.

I got to know Winnie well after that, and I soon found out that she was a lovely lady with a great sense of humour. I had lots of bed baths from Winnie, just as she had promised, and she cheered me up a lot. Life was a lot more interesting and fun suddenly. I just had to conquer one last hurdle – learning to walk again.

The 3rd October turned out to be a red letter day. Mr Lloyd Roberts, the esteemed surgeon, came to visit me on the ward. He was followed, as usual, by a gaggle of medical students. 'Hello again, Antony,' he greeted me. 'You have finally got through it all. Well done you!'

He began to talk to the group of students about my condition and all the operations and other medical procedures I had been through, while his secretary took lots of notes. Then the doctor turned his attention to me again.

'Right, Antony,' he said. 'Can you sit up and take big breaths for me, please? That's it – deep breath...and relax! And can you bend your knee now, please? Do it slowly, though'.

'I would like to try to stand up now,' I said, 'If that is alright with you?'

'Well, yes,' he said, seeming quite taken aback. 'If you think you could manage it'.

The nurses helped me out of bed, and I managed to

stand up alone. I felt like a telegraph pole, stretched out tall and thin. The doctor and the medical students were all very impressed. 'Can I try to walk now?' I asked.

Mr Lloyd Roberts acquiesced, and I managed to walk a few steps. The doctor was very surprised. He recommended more physiotherapy then, to continue to strengthen my legs.

The next week, matters continued to progress well. I had gained weight by now, and did not look so painfully skinny. One sunny day a nurse asked, 'Antony, would you like me to take you out in a wheelchair to get some fresh air? We could go around the Tadworth Court grounds'.

'Yes, please!' I replied. The nurse wheeled me around the gardens, and down to a nearby pig farm.

'Yeuch!' I exclaimed. 'That smells disgusting!'

'No worse than you smelt when you came out of your plaster cast,' the nurse replied, and we both laughed. I felt so happy that day, perhaps because life had become so much easier and more enjoyable now that I was free of the plaster cast. I'd endured a lot, and I really felt that now the only possible way was up.

The nurse took me to the stable yard nearby, and we went into a small building where visiting parents could buy refreshments and sit and relax when necessary. She brought me a cup of tea and some biscuits.

Just then an ambulance arrived in the nearby car park. I realised that the vehicle must have come from Great Ormond Street when I saw a boy being taken out of it on a stretcher. He was covered in plaster, just as I had been. I felt very sorry for him, and for his parents, who were following close behind the stretcher, presumably over to ward ZMA.

I spoke to the nurse about how sad this made me feel. 'But this is how Tadworth Court works,' she explained. 'You will soon be discharged, and others will take your place here. There will be a lot more children covered in plaster, and then they too will get better and go home and others will take their place'.

A thought struck me. 'Guess what, nurse?' I said to her. 'I just had a cup of tea without using my special straw!'

'I know, Antony,' she replied. 'And you opened your own packet of biscuits too, for the first time in weeks'.

I was so pleased, but also wistful, because I knew that my time at Tadworth Court would soon be drawing to a close. When we got back to the ward, the physiotherapist was waiting for me. She was holding a pair of wooden crutches. 'It's time for you to walk along the arched pathways,' she smiled.

We began immediately. Two nurses helped me out of the wheelchair, and handed me the crutches. I then walked alongside the physiotherapist, along the pathway. I was surprised how fast we progressed. I loved walking, and I felt as if I never wanted to stop. My legs and back felt as if they were becoming stronger by the minute.

Then I sat for a rest, on a bench seat near the beautiful flower beds. Suddenly, the physiotherapist called out in alarm. 'Why are you crying, Antony? Are you in pain?'

'No,' I said sadly.

'Please tell me what is wrong,' she begged.

'I don't want to go home yet,' I cried. 'I am going to miss this place. It's so beautiful!'

'But just think,' she said. 'Soon you will see all your friends, and you will be able to go back to school'.

'I don't want to go back to school,' I told her. I have been away for so long, and I won't be able to catch up with the school work'.

I could not be consoled, and when I got back to the ward I stayed in the cubicle on my own, listening to music on the radio. I could not seem to snap out of the gloom. At supper time I walked to the play room, using my crutches, to eat with the other children. After supper the Sister called me to her office.

'Antony,' she said, 'I have good news for you. Tomorrow you are going to be discharged from the hospital for good. Your Mum and Dad will be coming to take you home'.

I must not have looked impressed at this news, because she continued to speak. 'A little bird told me that you don't want to go home,' she said. 'I can help you with that if you like. I can put you back in plaster again'.

I had to laugh at that. 'Not in a million years!' I cried out.

'I'm glad to see that you have changed your tune,' smiled

the Sister.

I started to feel excited then about going home, but by the next morning I was in tears again. I didn't want to leave all the nurses, who I now considered to be my friends. In particular, I had become close to one nurse, Maggie Tamplin, who was just a little taller than me.

I had breakfast in my cubicle for the last time then, and all I had to do was wait for my parents to collect me. They were due some time before lunch, but I had not been told exactly when. A nurse came into the cubicle and handed me an envelope. I looked at her blankly. 'It's a birthday card,' she said. The Sister stood by her. 'That's right,' she told me. 'It's your birthday next week, on the 17th October'.

I was shocked, because I had completely forgotten about my birthday. 'It's probably because you have been in the hospital for so long,' said the nurse. I looked on a calendar then, and realised that I had been in hospital for seventy-five days – a very long time indeed! And now in just a few days I would be fifteen years old.

Mum and Dad finally arrived to collect me, and we all went into the ward office to speak to the Sister before we left. 'Antony, you won't be able to go back to school just yet,' she told me. 'You will need to work on your strength, and also take plenty of rest. Mr Lloyd Roberts says it would be best if you wait until the New Year to go back. Until then your headteacher, Mr Cotton, has arranged for you to have home tuition'.

She paused. 'And one other thing,' she added. ' I just want to tell you that you are the bravest teenager I have ever had in this ward'.

I was very proud when she said that, but I was also heartbroken to leave the hospital. I had become accustomed to being there, and despite the pain I had experienced within its walls, I had come to see it as a wonderful and magical place.

Before we left I went into my cubicle alone for one last time. It may sound odd, but I have to admit that I kissed my bed to say goodbye to it! Then my parents and I had to say goodbye and thank you to all the people who had looked after me.

The nurses and the sister gathered round Dad's car and watched me get in the back. 'I am so pleased that you can walk again,' a nurse told me. 'Nobody will have to lift you up to put you into that car ever again'.

The tears were streaming down my face as we prepared to leave. 'I am going to miss you all so much,' I said. 'I don't know how to thank you enough, for helping me to get through the difficult times. You are truly kind people, and complete professionals, and I will never forget you for as long as I live. Goodbye!'

And the 'Goodbyes' they called out in return seemed to echo in my head for ages as Dad slowly drove down the grand driveway and I left Tadworth Court for the final time.

Back at home, I felt subdued. My fifteenth birthday was approaching, but I was not as excited as I would usually have been. I suppose this was partly due to the fact that birthdays are not as exciting as you get older, but it was also because I was having serious emotional difficulties. I was filled with anxiety, and I could not figure out why

– I just seemed to have lost a lot of confidence in myself, and also I had lost interest in what was going on around me.

I did not want to see my friends – I didn't want to go to their houses, or to have them come around to visit me. The way I was feeling seemed to be connected to my school work. I was devastated and embarrassed by the fact that my mental ability seemed to have gone downhill – since I had been at Tadworth Court I could not read, write or spell any more, or even do simple sums. I felt that my friends would laugh at me and shun me because of this fact.

I got it into my head that I wanted to go back to Tadworth and live there – I really did not want to be in my own home any more. I felt guilty about this, and so I just stayed inside and kept myself to myself, watching the television and listening to the radio and not interacting with anybody. Except for my Mum and Dad of course – they took the brunt of my low mood. I couldn't seem to control myself and make an effort to be nice even to them, although I wanted to.

On my fifteenth birthday, my Mum organised a party and invited all my school friends. They came over and had a great time – but I found all the excitement too much. I was overwhelmed, and broke down in tears. Mum realised that I was struggling, and asked my friends nicely to go home. I felt awful about this, but they didn't seem to hold it against me, they just went off cheerfully, telling me not to worry and that they were sure that I would feel better soon. I was lucky to have such good friends!

One morning Mum decided that I needed some fresh air,

and that she would take me out for a stroll. I found it hard to walk with my crutches, so Mum hired a wheelchair from the Red Cross, and pushed me around the shops in nearby Purewell Cross. The wheelchair was hard for her to control though, especially when she had to cross the road - she struggled to get the chair back up onto the pavement.

Out of the blue, a man approached and helped Mum. 'I've seen your son in the local paper,' he told her. 'I read about how he bought a guide dog for the blind'.

'That's nice,' replied Mum. 'Thanks so much for helping us'.

'No problem,' he replied. 'In fact, I would like to arrange for Antony to have an electric wheelchair, if you think that would help him. He could be more independent then'.

'That sounds fantastic,' said my Mum. 'How much would it cost?'

'Don't worry about that,' he said. 'I am a member of a charity called TOC.H and we arrange loans of electric wheelchairs, free of charge'.

Mum gave him our address, and he promised to bring the wheelchair soon and show me how to use it. To our amazement he had arrived at our house with the wheelchair before we even got home from the shops – he was outside waiting for us!

I really liked the electric wheelchair – it looked cool and it turned out to be immense fun to drive. I steered it with a joy stick, and I could go left or right, backwards or forwards. It was powered by a big battery. When the battery was fully charged I would know, because I could see that the beads inside had risen to the top – when the beads dropped, this indicated that the battery was low. It was a fantastic mobility gadget!

Mum asked the man how long we could borrow the wheelchair for, and he said as long as necessary. It certainly did help me – I went all over town in it, and I started to enjoy life a lot more. We kept it until the end of January, by which time I was back on my feet properly. Even now I often think of the man from TOC.H and how lucky we were to meet him on our trip to the shops that day!

In November I started home tuition. Mr Cotton from Twynham had organised this, as he had promised before I went into hospital. Two kind ladies came to my house to work with me. I had to read a lot, and I found this difficult. The words all seemed very long, and quite incomprehensible. I also did not find it easy to write or spell. I hated Maths too, and resented being made to learn how to do all these things. I was not a well-behaved student!

I liked History and Geography more than the other subjects though. One day in the tuition session, one of the teachers was checking my knowledge. 'Many hundreds of years ago Antony', she said, 'The farmers had to cut down a lot of trees to make way for something. What was that?'

I was in a bad mood that day. 'I don't know,' I said grumpily.

'Oh you do, Antony, she insisted. 'We talked a lot about

it the other day, and I showed you in your history book. Come on now, concentrate. The farmers hundreds of years ago had to make space for what?'

'The farmers..' I said slowly, ' Hundreds of years ago. Had to cut down the trees to make space for a .. a bl****y motorway!'

The teacher couldn't help laughing, but when she finally stopped she shook her head at me. 'No,' she said. 'Crops'.

My tutors gave me no option – I had to work with them to catch up. This perseverance paid off, and my reading did gradually improve. I still struggled a lot with Maths and English though, especially handwriting, which I found very slow and painful because my hands had swollen with arthritis. I could not keep the pen comfortably in my grip.

But the tutors kept visiting, and I knew I had to push myself, because I did not want all their efforts to go to waste. I had three months of school work to catch up on, which was a lot. And in between the school work I had to find time to do my exercises. I had to walk a lot to strengthen my muscles, and learn to move my back properly. I also had to find time for lots of long hot baths to soak my legs and ease all the aches and pains I was feeling. One day after my bath I realised that my skin tone was normal again, and that all the flaked rough skin on my legs had disappeared. I was very relieved.

Just two days before Christmas a new problem surfaced. I felt hot and unwell, but when Mum checked I did not have a temperature. I itched all over though, and the skin all over my body was bright red. Mum called Dr

Cantlie and he came to see me.

'Don't worry, Antony,' he said, 'This is all to do with the fact that you were in plaster for so long. Now that the dead skin has gone, the air on the new skin is making you feel itchy'. He wrote a prescription for some cream, and then continued. 'I am so pleased to see that you are walking more,' he said. 'How is your school tuition progressing?'

'My reading is getting better,' I told him, 'But my Maths and spelling ability is a disaster'.

'Don't worry about it Antony,' said the doctor. 'I am sure you will improve in time'.

Before Dr Cantlie left, he had a look at my knee, and he was very pleased to see that the two big lumps of bone had been removed from my femur. When he had gone, Mum went off to get the cream that he had prescribed. As soon as she came back I rubbed the cream onto my body, and the itching eased almost immediately. It was a great relief.

Christmas Day dawned, and as usual we were up early, opening our presents. Pickles the poodle ripped the wrapping paper to shreds as he always did. Mum and Dad cooked the Christmas lunch together – turkey with all the trimmings – and we had Mum's delicious home-made Christmas pudding for dessert. And of course, we went to Ashtree House later in the afternoon, for Grandad's traditional Christmas tea party. It was a wonderful day, as family Christmasses always were.

On Boxing Day I had a wonderful outing. I was picked up by Mr Staniforth, the Mayor of Christchurch, and his special Scout, in his black Daimler, and we all went off together to Mudeford Quay to see the Mudeford Lifeboat Carnival. I felt as if I was royalty that day. It was a very special event – the Quay was crowded with onlookers, many of them in fancy dress.

The Mayor introduced me to many people at the Lifeboat Station, and I really had a brilliant time with him. I felt that he was such a kind and thoughtful man to do this for me, and I was really grateful.

Now Christmas was over, and 1973 was on its way out. It had been a terrible year, but at last it was over, and I could move on.

Chapter Fourteen
School, Scouts and the Piano

In the first week of January 1974, I returned to school. On my first day back, at school assembly, Mr Cotton greeted me and asked whether I would like to say a few words to all my fellow pupils, and to the staff. I stood on the stage, in front of hundreds of children and all the teachers, all looking at me, but for some reason, I did not feel even the slightest twinge of nerves as I began to speak.

First I thanked Mr Cotton for welcoming me back. Then I started to tell everyone all about Tadworth Court. I told them about the wonderful nurses and doctors who had cared for me, and about what a fantastic place Tadworth was. Then I told them more personal things – it all came flooding out, more than I had intended to say.

'I was terrified of the operation,' I said. 'I thought that would be the worst part, and when it was over things would improve. But when I woke up from the anaesthetic, I found myself trapped in a full body plaster, like a turtle'. Some of the children laughed at that.

'It sounds funny, but it wasn't,' I told them. 'I felt claustrophobic, trapped on my back in bed. I was scared, homesick, and lonely. There were plenty of other children in the same predicament as me, or worse, and I felt so sorry for them. Some of them never seemed to have visitors, and I knew I was lucky that my family came to see me so often'. The faces of the children in front of me looked more serious then.

'It was really hard,' I went on. 'There were some

moments when I thought I could not cope with the hardship. I even thought about taking my own life'. Mr Cotton seemed very concerned to hear this, and some of the other teachers looked quite emotional too. I struggled on with my speech.

'I was worried about my family too,' I said. 'My Mum and Dad looked so tired when they came to see me. I felt so guilty about that. I honestly didn't think I would get through at times.'

'I missed school too – I love Twynham,' I said truthfully. 'And I missed all my friends. But somehow, I did get through the difficult times, and one day the plaster came off, and suddenly I felt a lot more free, and a lot happier. And so here I am, back at school again!'

Mr Cotton spoke then. 'How do you feel about being back at school, Antony?' he asked.

'Well,' I replied, 'I got to the point where, once I was out of plaster, I actually did not want to leave the hospital. I had begun to appreciate what a special and precious place Tadworth Court was, with its beautiful gardens, and all the caring people who worked there. By the time I left, it was a real wrench. But I am glad now to see all my friends again. I have learned resilience, I think – that life does change, and some things are beyond our control. But that we can cope with change and learn from it and that, if we hold firm, in the end everything will turn out fine'.

My speech was over. The headteacher thanked me profusely. 'I think we can all learn a lot from Antony,' he said, 'And from his attitude to life. Antony has learned to overcome hardship and to work with difficulties instead of fighting them. If and when any of you children face hardship in the lives ahead of you, I want you to think back to this day, and take courage from the lesson he has taught you'.

Mr Cotton then asked the children if they wanted to ask me any questions about my time in hospital, and lots of them did. Their questions were mainly about the sort of food we were given, and whether we could watch as much television as we wanted while we were in hospital! Everybody seemed interested in my answers. Then I sat down while Mr Cotton finished the assembly. I had enjoyed my few minutes in the spotlight, but I was not sorry that it was over.

Now I had to get on with school life. The practicalities were not easy – I had to move from room to room for each lesson, and that was slow going on my crutches. Mr Cotton assigned one of my friends to help – he came with me wherever I went, and carried the briefcase which held all my school books, which meant that both of us were late for our lessons! Eventually the teachers agreed that I should leave each lesson early, with my friend, to avoid the rush in the corridors between classes and ensure that I got to my next lesson in time.

The problems I had with my school work were tougher to sort out. I was really struggling - I had lost a lot of confidence, and although my friends did their best to lift my mood and help me along, I was frustrated at myself for not doing as well in lessons as I would have liked. The teachers were very patient with me, but it was still a struggle.

My academic subjects had changed now. I no longer studied History or Geography, but I still did English and

Maths. (I hated Maths, but it was compulsory for everyone). I also took Art, Music, Biology, General Science and Domestic Science. And I did another subject, known as Project. Although I am often told that I have a good memory (and I have kept a lot of school reports and other mementoes from my younger days) I cannot remember for the life of me what that project was all about!

The main reason I found the school work so hard was because my back was causing me a lot of pain. I was pleased that I now stood so straight, but I was not accustomed to it. All my muscles were working hard to maintain their new positions, and it hurt to walk.

In PE, I was allowed to sit on the sidelines. I liked watching the cricket, rugby and football outside – and whenever the football came near me I would give it a good kick back into the game, although I knew I was not supposed to! I just wanted to feel that I was a part of things.

I liked watching the basketball best – this took place indoors in the gym, and I was allowed to keep score. This helped me to keep track of the game and made me feel that I was properly involved. PE had never been one of my favourite activities anyhow (apart from football) so I didn't feel as though I was missing out.

Back at home, I had given up trying to play the cornet, since the embarrassment of attempting to do so at the Tadworth Summer Fayre and finding that I had run out of puff. I still loved music though, and used to sneak off to play Grandad's piano at Ashtree House.

Grandad wanted me to play the cornet, not the piano,

and would often try to persuade me to do so. But it was the piano I wanted, and I taught myself to play on it. I had a good ear, although I never learned to read music, and I soon learned to pick out tunes. Greensleeves was my favourite.

One day I arrived at Ashtree, and found that the lid of the piano had been locked. Grandad clearly did not want me to play today! He had gone out, so I couldn't speak to him about it. The housekeeper was there though, and she offered to help. 'Your Grandad's gone to work,' she said. 'You can have a quick play while he is out. The key in his study, in a small box inside his roll-top desk'.

I found the key, unlocked the lid of the piano, and played to my heart's content. Suddenly the housekeeper burst in. 'Your Grandad's back!' she exclaimed. 'Quick, lock the piano and put the key back in the study!'

I did as she told me as fast as I could, then rushed back, and by the time Grandad came into the room I was standing innocently looking out of the window, while the housekeeper dusted the piano nearby. He looked at us sharply, but said nothing.

The next day, I repeated this performance – went into Ashtree House while Grandad was out, played on the piano, and then returned the key to the box in his desk. This time, as soon as he came home, he called me into the hallway to speak to him. 'You haven't been playing my piano have you?' he asked, with a glint in his eye.

'No, Grandad,' I said. 'I would like to, but I can't because the lid is locked'.

The next morning when I arrived at Ashtree House, Grandad was home. He called me into the sun lounge where he sat drinking coffee with my parents and some of the riding school workers.

'Antony has a confession to make,' he announced.

My heart beat fast in my chest. 'Have I?' I asked nervously.

'You have,' he confirmed. 'You have been playing on my piano without permission. Am I right or am I wrong?'

'No, I really haven't,' I squeaked in dismay. How could he possibly have guessed? I wondered to myself.

'Come with me,' Grandad said to the assembled group, and we all trooped after him into the piano room. He was clearly enjoying this.

'Now,' he said. 'I believe that you went into the study, found the key, and used it to unlock the piano when I was out, then after you had played you returned the key, and thought I would never know,' he said.

I kept quiet. 'You made one mistake, Antony,' Grandad said. 'You don't like horses, do you?'

'What on earth has that got to do with it?' I exclaimed.

'Well,' he said. 'I suspected that someone had been tampering with my things. So I put a piece of horsehair over the piano keys – and you snapped the hair when you played, providing me with proof that my suspicions were correct'.

Grandad held the broken pieces of horse hair up to the assembled crowd and they all burst out laughing. He spoke to the housekeeper then, 'Did you, or did you not, aid and abet Antony in his crime?'

'I did, Sir,' she admitted. 'Then you shall both be banished from Ashtree House for a whole week,' he declared – but then, seeing her shocked face, he assured her that he was only joking. 'I missed my vocation in life,' he said. 'I should have been a detective. Antony, of course you can play the piano from now on – all you have to do is ask first!'

Everyone went off about the riding school then, and I stayed behind with Grandad. He looked at me and smiled. 'I'll get my own back, young man,' he said, 'Just you wait and see!'

I continued to play the piano at Ashtree House, and made good progress. One day, I told my music teacher at school how I loved to play Greensleeves, and he asked whether I would play in front of the school. 'Just before the Easter Holidays, we will have a music concert,' he said. 'It would be great if you would agree to play your piece then'.

I agreed readily and soon the day of the concert arrived. I felt well prepared. A few people performed before me, and when it was my turn the teacher introduced me, 'Next, we have a very special boy,' he said, 'Who is going to play us a beautiful piece of music'.

I came out from behind the curtain to the sound of applause. I was on the stage, and I looked down to see Mum, Dad and Grandad sitting together in the front row of the audience. I bowed, and took my seat at the piano.

The school orchestra struck up, to signal that it was time for me to begin.

I raised my hands, lowered them to the piano...and froze in mid air. I was confused, because my hands just would not move further down. When I tried to force them, I began to shake. 'Are you alright, Antony?' asked my teacher, but I couldn't reply. I seemed to have lost the power of speech.

Minutes passed, but they seemed like hours. I looked towards the audience, then back towards the piano, and still my hands refused to move. I looked up at the music teacher in panic. 'Don't worry, Antony,' he said kindly. 'You are experiencing stage fright. This often happens to performers, and it is nothing to be concerned about'.

It did help to put a name to my condition, but I still couldn't play the piece. I was very disappointed in myself and just wanted to run off the stage, hide and cry. I didn't though. I made myself get up and walk to the front of the stage. 'I am very sorry,' I told the audience. 'I am suffering from stage fright, and I simply cannot bring myself to play a single note. I am so sorry to disappoint you all'.

To my surprise, everybody applauded, and I bowed in response. As I did so, I glanced down towards where my family sat, and was surprised to see that although Mum and Dad looked concerned, Grandad was smiling serenely.

In the car on the way home, Grandad was gloating. 'I told you I'd get my own back,' he said. 'I knew that you'd freeze in front of an audience. Now, are you going to give up the darned piano and get on and play the cornet again?'

'On your bike, Grandad!' I responded, and he chuckled all the way back, until we dropped him off at Ashtree House.

It was the Easter Holidays now. Although I was still on crutches, the weather was fine and I was allowed outside to play with my friends again. I had been desperate to ride my American Spider bike, but it was not as easy as I had hoped – I still had to build up my stamina.

One day I was playing outside with a group of friends, and looked over the road towards my house. Suddenly a feeling of sadness came over me. I imagined that I could see myself on the inside of the house looking out, as the others played without me. All the time that I was inside I had longed to join my friends on the street but now that I was here as I had hoped, I still didn't feel that I was fully a part of things. I knew that part of me would always be separate, different. I had to struggle to hold the tears back.

'Come on mate,' said my friend, pulling me back into the game. 'You're dwelling on the past again, aren't you?' I don't know how he had guessed, but he was right, and I knew that he had made a good point. I needed to concentrate on what was happening here and now, and not keep drifting back into the past.

I was soon distracted by an offer to join the local Boy Scout group. The leader was my friend's father, and the Scout Hut was in Mallory Close, near our old house on the Somerford Estate. My friend's Dad told my parents and I that the Scouts were good for building boys' confidence, so I decided to give it a try.

I liked Scouts right away. A lot of my old Junior School friends attended the group. I was worried at first because I was told I would have to learn the Scout Law, 'A Scout is to be trusted. A Scout is loyal. A Scout is friendly and considerate...' There was a long list of the necessary qualities one needed to become a Scout and I was concerned that I would not be able to memorise them all. Fortunately by dint of repetition all the words eventually seeped into my brain, and I can still remember them today!

After I had learned to repeat the Scout Law, I was allowed to wear the uniform. My Mum took me to a special uniform shop in Christchurch to buy it - black trousers and a dark green shirt, with a Scout badge on the front pocket, a brown leather belt with a silver buckle, and a green beret with another badge on. We all wore burgundy neckerchiefs fastened with brown woggles. I really felt the business when I was dressed up in my Scout outfit – very important and worthy, as if I was a soldier in the army!

Apart from having fun, we were taught practical skills, such as knot tying. I only ever managed to tie a reef knot (which sometimes turned itself into a Granny knot) – my fingers were too small to attempt the others. We also each made ourselves a 'Monkey's fist'. This was a fantastic piece of equipment – a ball of nylon rope attached to another six feet of rope cord. It could be used as a lasso, or to help climb trees. Or you could make it into a belt with the ball as a buckle (crochet was taught for this purpose, and I turned out to be good at it).

No Scout would have been without his Monkey's fist in those days – although now it would be considered a complete hazard on the grounds of Health and Safety! We also each had a Scout issue sheath knife, and we were taught how to use it safely and sensibly – I can't imagine that knives would be allowed as standard Scout equipment nowadays either.

It was soon 'Bob a Job' week – so-called because we earned a bob, or a shilling, for every job we undertook out in the community. We had to go around our local area, asking if anybody needed any jobs doing, 'Bob a job?' we would ask. If a household gave us a job, we would give them a sticker in return. The sticker said that they'd already been 'Bob a jobbed' so that no other Scouts would knock and ask for the rest of the week!

Scouts still carry out this activity today, although now it is known as 'Scout Community Week'. My competitive streak came out here, and I worked very hard to raise as much money as I could. Grandad and Uncle Matt helped by giving me loads of work at Ashtree House. I mucked out the stables, swept out the yard, helped to feed the horses and to clean the tack. I was constantly busy, and for every job I did, I got paid a shilling.

By the end of the week I was pleased to discover that I had raised more money than any other Scout. The Scout Master gave me a community badge and a large cup. The funds went towards paying for a new scout hut, and also for our camping trip, which was set to be in July.

I was really excited about camping, as it was the first time I had been away with the Scouts. The camp would last for a week, although I was only going to be allowed to join in for the weekend, because I wasn't able to join in with some of the activities. I couldn't wait though – it felt good to have something to look forward to.

Meanwhile, the new term had started and back at Twynham I was settling back down to my school work. I had started to feel much happier and stronger by now. There was only one blight on the horizon – I didn't have hot school meals, but took sandwiches, and my Mum seemed determined that I should have more impressive packed lunches than anybody else in the school. (Maybe I'd inherited my competitive streak from her!)

Every day Mum would put something new and different in my lunch. There was far too much – I couldn't eat it all – and what was worse was that the other children constantly took the mickey out of me for my 'posh' sandwiches. The limit came on the day where, on top of all the usual food, she gave me a chicken leg – with salt and pepper cruets so I could season it! The other kids had a field day with this. However, I soon turned the situation to my advantage. I figured out that their mockery was caused by jealousy, and that they would have given anything for such delicious lunches. So I offered my food for sale – anything that I couldn't eat went to the highest bidder.

My coffers soon swelled. The money jar in my bedroom was bursting, by the time Mum noticed and asked where all the money was coming from. She laughed when I told her what I'd been up to, but took notice then when I asked her not to overdo it with the packed lunch. I was happy with cheese and crackers, a piece of fruit and a Wagon Wheel, which was all that I got after that!

One of my favourite subjects at school was Domestic Science. I cooked with Mum at home – she was a dab hand in the kitchen – which gave me a head start. In the school classroom I learned new skills – one day we cooked breakfast, which was all fried, including the bacon, eggs, mushrooms, bread and tomatoes.

I was a success in the school kitchen. One day I made a wonderful Madeira cake – it looked like a work of art. When I got it home I ate far more than my share though, and ended up with a severe bout of diarrhoea. When I see a Madeira cake even now I can't help thinking of it as a 'Diarrhoea cake'!

Another day, the cookery teacher asked the class to each make a dessert. 'Choose something that people would eat for dessert at an expensive restaurant' she said. I looked through the recipe book, and was entranced by the picture of the raspberry souffle. I wanted to make something really impressive.

The teacher was doubtful when I showed her my choice. 'It is very complicated, and very expensive,' she warned. 'I am agreeable, if you are sure you want to try it, but you will have to check with your mother first'.

Mum sent me in for the next domestic science lesson armed with all the ingredients to make a large raspberry souffle. I had lemons, gelatine, double cream and whipping cream – and fresh raspberries, of course, sourced from Grandad's fruit and vegetable business.

The teacher worked with me to make the raspberry souffle, and it turned out wonderfully. It was huge, rose to be even bigger, and the fresh raspberries on top made it look very professional. I was really proud, especially when I looked around at the work of my classmates, who had all cooked quite ordinary desserts. I carried it carefully home.

Mum 'oohed' and 'aahed' over my dessert, as I had hoped. But then she said, 'Antony, I have to ask you a question. Why did you make that particular pudding, when you are allergic to raspberries?'

My bubble burst then. I had been so carried away with the success of my grand project that I had forgotten all about my raspberry allergy! I did manage a few spoonfuls though – the dessert was delicious, and the rest of my family were more than pleased to finish it off.

It was summer now, and boiling hot in the school buildings and on the playing grounds. The end of year exams came and went, and again I was pleased to find out that I had done reasonably well. I had failed my English and Maths exams, but my teachers acknowledged that I tried hard and had made some progress. I had done well in my Project work (the teacher noted in my report that I had involved myself completely in my visits and had produced a good folder. I do wish I could remember what that Project was!)

I did quite well in my other subjects too – but it was becoming clear by now that I was pulling ahead in Art. I think I was starting to work out for myself already what I was good at, and gravitating towards it. My report that year states that I had an eye for structure and made very good observational drawings. I was certainly heading towards the realisation that I would have a career in Art.

The Summer holidays began, and it was time for the Scouts camping trip. I had hoped to be allowed to stay for the whole week after all, but I was told it would only be possible to stay the weekend as had been planned, mainly because it was very hard for me to get around the field on my crutches.

We set up camp in a big open field near Hurn Airport, in Christchurch, and I will always remember the noise of the planes coming in to land and taking off nearby. I slept in a big brown canvas Ridge tent with five or six other Scouts. Unfortunately it was not waterproof – it had not been properly waxed, and so the rain came in and soaked us all, and our possessions, gradually through over the weekend.

The other boys played tricks on me, but I didn't mind, it was all part of the fun. One day, they sent me off to ask the Scout Master for a left-handed screwdriver. I was puzzled when instead of answering me he headed straight over to the nearby group of giggling boys and told them off! One of them explained to me later that there was no such thing as a left-handed screwdriver.

The first night we had a big camp fire, and sat around it singing. I didn't much like the songs – they were old-fashioned and boring, and reminded me of when I first joined the Bournemouth Silver Band and had to spend hours practising 'Oklahoma'. The Ging Gang Goolie song was my least favourite of them all – I thought that the Scout experience would be greatly improved if they had some decent music. The Ying Tong song would have been much better, I thought, but I didn't dare to recommend it.

That weekend we were all taught how to light a small camp fire and use our knives to carve out wooden tent pegs. The other boys cooked, but I was not allowed to help. I was only permitted to peel potatoes. When I saw the size of the cooking pot I realised why I had been told that it was too dangerous for me to cook – the pan was much too heavy for me to lift, and so big I could almost have fallen into it and been cooked myself!

I joined in a lot of the games, but could only watch when they used their compasses to follow a treasure trail. Both nights I slept soundly, and was only woken by the bugle call for breakfast. On the day I was due to leave, we had to tidy the tent ready for inspection.

The Scout Master scoured the tent, and one of my friends got into serious trouble because an adult magazine was found under the mattress of his camp bed. Suddenly I froze. The Scout Master had called my name, and he did not sound happy. He was looking inside my camping bag. 'Oh dear,' he said, 'What have we got here Antony?'

I racked my brains. What could I have packed that I wasn't allowed to bring? Then he suddenly stopped rummaging. 'I'm sorry,' he said quietly. He had found my spare pair of surgical shoes – I had not put them under my camp bed because I had not wanted the others to see them and laugh at them. I didn't mind – I was just pleased not to have been caught with an adult magazine!

My Dad was due to collect me later, but before I went a friend of mine took me aside. A small orange tent was set up next to the large one that we had been sleeping in, with a sign attached saying, 'Do not disturb. Lady Scout Leader unwell inside'. Our Scout master had warned us to take care to be quiet around the tent, especially at night time, and we had been tiptoeing around it for the last two days.

'That lady has been in there all weekend,' said my friend. 'Do you think we should check in case she has died of her illness?' Our Scout Master was nowhere to be seen, so we gingerly crept up to the tent, unzipped it and peered inside. There was nothing and nobody in there, except a piece of paper lying on the groundsheet. We picked it up curiously. 'Gotcha!' it read. There never had been a sick lady in the tent – it was just a ploy our Scout Master had devised to make sure we weren't too noisy at night time!

Dad arrived to take me home then, and I said goodbye to everyone. I hoped that another time I would be able to camp for longer, as I had really enjoyed myself.

The rest of the holidays soon passed. To earn extra pocket money I helped with the chores at Ashtree House. My cousin and I did the mowing, taking turns with the large petrol mower. One day, my cousin started the mower and left me to carry on alone, saying that he would soon be back. The mower stopped soon after, so I decided to start it myself. I had to stand on top to pull the lever using a cord, but it still would not start. So I fiddled with the motor a little – and all of a sudden the mower took off, with me still standing on top of it. I managed to jump off, but the machine was out of control and ran amok in Grandad's flower beds, dead-heading his roses well before they were ready! Grandad was extremely cross about all this, but fortunately my cousin and I still got paid for our work.

It was the World Cup again this summer, and I had high hopes that Brazil would win again. However, it was not to be – West Germany got the cup, and Brazil came a disappointing fourth. I was still determined to support them in the future though.

September came, and the new term started – the

beginning of my final year at Twynham! I had just four subjects to concentrate on for my CSE exams – English, Maths, Biology and Art.   I also studied Home and Community, but there was no examination for this subject.

I had my 16th birthday in October. It was funny to think of all the things I could now legally do – smoke and drink, even get married with my parent's permission! None of this particularly appealed to me though – I liked to lead a clean and healthy life, so smoking and drinking were out of the question. And somehow I didn't think I was likely to get married in the year ahead, given that I didn't have a girlfriend!

Chapter Fifteen
Fun and Games

I was still with the Scouts. One December night at 9pm, after the Scout meeting finished, I went night fishing with some of my school friends. We met at Mudeford Harbour very late at night, kitted out with warm clothing and Tilley lamps for warmth and light, and well-furnished with provisions. There were six or seven of us. Most of the others smoked by now, although their parents didn't know it, so they were puffing away (although of course I didn't). It felt exciting to be out so late.

We cast our lines, and sat to wait in the dark. And wait. We sat all night without a single pull on those lines. It was only when morning came that we realised we had been caught out by odd December tides. The sea had retreated during the night, so we had been sitting watching lines that lay stranded on the sand. The bait was still attached. We were frozen to the bones and mightily embarrassed, but we had to laugh.

At school and home, I paid a lot of attention to my drawing. I knew by now that I had the potential for a career in art and design. I went out a fair bit with my friends (often to the cinema) but most of my spare time was spent drawing. The old lady next door took a great interest in my work – she was disabled too; she'd had a leg amputated. I would take my portfolio round to show her, and we would chat about it and about art in general.

I was good at copying architectural drawings, especially brickwork. I liked cartoons and animation too, although the art teachers at school did not encourage this. I could also paint, and loved trying out new techniques. The more I did, the more inspired I became, and I looked forward to leaving school and concentrating even more on my artwork. My dream was now to become a professional artist.

Christmas was looming, and the school holidays began. That year the Scouts had a Christmas Fair at the hut. To my surprise I was put in charge of the whole event, as the Scoutmaster realised that I'd had a lot of experience of fund-raising in all my charity work, raising funds for the Guide Dog Association. We raised £90 in total – a very good amount for those days.

Soon the holidays were over, and it was time to go back to Twynham to start a new term of school again. All my friends had started to ride motorbikes to school now that they had turned sixteen, and Uncle Matt didn't want me to be left out. Most of my friends had Japanese bikes – made by Honda, Yamaha, Suzuki or Kawasaki. It was a new world opening up for teenagers and adults, as the Japanese motor industry flooded into the UK with their new cheap but quality products.

Unfortunately, most of us had no idea how to ride the bikes or how to use the roads safely, so it was also a rather dangerous time. In those days you could ride a bike on a provisional licence without taking a test, for up to two years, as long as the engine was less than 50cc in size. So Matt bought me an Italian moped – a Fantic – from Fantic Motors in Bournemouth.

I had no idea how to ride a bike, but I desperately wanted to be able to show off my new acquisition, and by dint of perseverance I got used to it in the end. In February I received my provisional licence, and proudly rode my bike to school for the first time, with two 'L' plates fitted to it.

My new bike was really cool, but also very noisy when I started it. The sound of the engine would reverberate up the street, especially on frosty mornings. It was great! The bike had a rack on the back wheel frame, onto which I would tie my briefcase with strong bungee ropes. I would rev the engine and speed all the way up to school.

I couldn't park the bike at the school, though, because it was impossible to lock it. There was no ignition key – the bike started simply by kick-starting the engine and revving. So to keep the bike safe from vandals or thieves, I left it in the driveway of a friend's house – luckily he lived just opposite Twynham School, in Sopers Lane.

One weekend, I rode my bike out with a group of friends, to Brockenhurst in the New Forest. We went to the water splash, which is at the entrance to the village. This was a ford, with running water. Sometimes, if it had rained heavily, it was too deep to pass through safely. It was deep that day, and most of us decided to take another route. One friend decided to take a chance though, and tried to drive through the ford. His engine soon seized up and stalled – and we, kind and thoughtful friends that we were, simply left him there to sort himself out. I suppose he must have eventually dried out or found help of some sort.

We were cruel in those days. One friend of ours had a Russian motorbike, a cheap one, and the others mocked him for it, saying that it was a girl's bike with pedals. It did look rather girly. We were all enjoying our ride out in the Forest though. But then some of my friends started playing up – doing wheelies and other silly stunts, which was dangerous on the main Forest roads. My friend with the Russian bike decided to go home early, and I said that I would go with him.

First we went off to the nearest petrol station to fill up our bikes ready for the journey home. We had ridden a lot of miles that day, and we realised that our tanks would be low. As we turned back towards home we passed the spot where we had left the rest of our group, and soon we caught up with them. They had run out of petrol and were slumped disillusioned next to their bikes. As we rode by they started kicking their bikes and swearing angrily.

I shouted at them as we passed, 'You guys should ride a girl's bike! At least it would get you home!' They chased us up the road then, shouting angrily, but of course they had no chance of catching up.

My friend laughed happily. 'Thank you for that, Antony,' he said. 'You have made my day. I owe you one'.

'You're welcome,' I said. We rode on. Soon we reached my friend's father's farm, on the border of the Forest, in Bransgore. We raced up the narrow country lane which led to the farmhouse. Suddenly I hit a pot hole, and was catapulted off my bike, did a somersault over the handlebars and landed head first in a cow pat.

At least it was a soft landing. But the cow pat was fresh and new, and left me stinking, with green and black skid marks all over my coat. It was horrid. My friend rushed over and helped me sit up – and I literally saw stars spinning around above my head!

We went into the farmhouse then, where his Dad cleaned me up, all the time tutting over how I had managed to get myself into such a predicament.

I had another big adventure not long after. My friend Garry came to visit one day and asked whether I would like to go fishing that evening, in Stanpit Marsh in Mudeford, with him and his brother and another friend. Of course, I said that I would love to.

We decided not to take our bicycles because of all the fishing gear we had to carry. It was a twenty-five minute walk to the bridge over the marsh which we had chosen to fish from. It was dark and cold, but all was going well, when suddenly my friend looked over his shoulder. 'Uh-oh,' he said, in a worried tone of voice. I followed his line of sight and realised what he was panicking about. While we had been intent on our task the tide had tricked us again. It had crept in behind us, and now we were totally surrounded by water and cut off from the path home.

The four of us realised that we needed to leave as soon as possible. My friends were concerned about me, as I was shorter than the others and had no Wellington boots to protect me from the water. Not that wellies would have helped me much – the water was up to two feet deep in places!

'Don't worry about me,' I said to the others, 'I'll be fine. Let's get going!'

We packed up quickly. The water was very deep and fast-running, and was still rising. So we set off, four of us in a line, each holding our fishing gear above our heads to protect it from the water. Eventually we reached another bridge further on. We were soaked, and felt really cold and miserable, so we stopped for a few minutes to take a breather. There was a full moon and we could see that the water was still rising.

A fisherman on a nearby boat caught sight of us and called out. 'Stop there on the bridge,' he called. 'You'll drown otherwise!'

But we kept going regardless. Just five hundred yards to go until we were safe... and so we struggled on, and made it, back at about ten pm. My parents were away at the time, and I was staying with my Grandad at Ashtree House. Luckily he'd had an early night, so he was fast asleep when I let myself in, and he had no idea what I had been up to, and how much danger I had been in.

Around that time I had a trip to Great Ormond Street Hospital to see Mr Lloyd Roberts at the Outpatient Department. I travelled up with my parents on the train. I remember that Mum had made a huge flask of vegetable soup, which we took with us. It was her speciality and I still remember how good it tasted – it was made with onions, swede, potatoes, garlic and an oxo cube, all liquidised into a soup. It was better than anything we could have bought in a restaurant.

Mr Lloyd Roberts asked how I was doing and what I had been up to. I told him enthusiastically all about my new Fantic bike and what fun I had on it, riding to and fro to school and going out with my friends. His jaw dropped in astonishment as he listened to me. 'You cannot ride a motorbike,' he said, 'It is simply out of the question. If at any time you have an accident and break any of your bones you could be hospitalised for months

– or you might never walk again. No motorbikes, do you understand me, Antony?'

I was really annoyed with myself for mentioning my bike, and upset that he had told me, in front of Mum and Dad, not to ride it any more. I realise now, though, that he was only acting out of concern – motorbikes are dangerous and I could have done myself a lot of damage if I had been involved in a road traffic accident.

The consultant then told me that my Great Ormond Street days were now over for good. I was sixteen years old – no longer a child – and therefore no longer qualified for treatment at the hospital. I had mixed feelings about this. I had bad memories of hospital – the pain and discomfort of being in plaster still haunted me - but I felt sad that I would no longer see the lovely nurses, or the other children that I had made friends with over the years.

In April that year my care was officially transferred over to Southampton General Hospital.   I had a new orthopaedic consultant now – Mr Wilkinson. He said that I was doing well, but emphasised the importance of exercise. I was to use a bicycle, he told me, to bend my legs and hips to promote flexibility, and to ward off arthritis. He seemed to have a good knowledge of my condition and so I trusted him, and listened carefully to his instructions.

Over the years I'd had various problems with my surgical shoes, which had to be made a distance from home, and still never seemed quite right. One day my Mum, frustrated with all these problems, got hold of the telephone directory and called around all the local shoemakers to see if she could find one who would make surgical shoes. She struck lucky in the end – she found a small firm in Boscombe, Bournemouth, who said that they could make the shoes, if she got a referral from the NHS.

So Mum arranged for the NHS to authorise this firm to make me a pair of shoes – and they came up trumps, with a really good pair, a perfect fit, made with soft brown leather. The shoemaker was very experienced and understanding. I was delighted – although I had to be very careful to take care of my shoes, as I was only allowed two pairs a year on the NHS. They made my life so much easier and more comfortable, and I was very grateful to that shoemaker, and to my Mum for taking matters into her own hands and sorting it all out for me.

I was starting to enjoy school more now. On Friday nights I would go out with a group of friends, to the '16+ Club' – a youth club held at the local Riverside Pub. This club was open to all the local schools, and was often very busy. One night when it was packed solid I was bullied by a group of boys, who kept pushing me and calling me 'Shorty'.

I tried to ignore them, but it was hard, especially when one of the oldest and toughest of them told me, 'You're not wanted here. It's a club for people aged sixteen and above, not for infants'.

I was really hurt, but determined to ignore them and rise above their taunting. My friends were becoming very annoyed, but I told them not to worry. I didn't want to be the cause of any trouble. Then, in the toilet, I got cornered by five of the boys. Their leader, the one who had called me an infant, told me to give him money if I wanted to be left alone.

I gave the boy a pound, which was all I had on me. When I came out of the toilets I told my friends what had happened and they were furious. They looked everywhere for those boys – but the bullies had already left.

The next day I was at Ashtree House with my Uncle Matt. I usually spent Saturday mornings there. He was interviewing candidates for a part-time job at the stables, and I was sitting in. I could not believe my eyes when I saw the first candidate – it was the bully from the night before! As soon as he saw me he turned as red as a beetroot.

'Hello,' I said calmly. 'How are you?'

'Um...Um....,' he was clearly panicking. He turned to my uncle. 'I've changed my mind about the job'.

'Why?' asked Matt, in confusion.

The boy looked all around, and it was clear that if he could have run away, he would, but there was no way to exit the room without pushing past Matt and myself.

I looked straight at him, enjoying my sweet moment of revenge. 'You might as well tell my Uncle the truth,' I said evenly. 'And by the way – you owe me a pound!'

Chapter Sixteen
A Testing Time

That spring I decided to leave the Scouts, because I needed to concentrate on my school work. Mock exams loomed, and I knew how important they were for my future prospects. I was worried how I would cope with long periods sitting in the hall, and how my hands would feel after hours of writing. I worried about all sorts of things, even about whether anyone would be able to read my handwriting on the exam papers.

As it turned out, though, the Mocks, which I took in May, did not go too badly. My teachers were pleased with my results, which I found encouraging. My House Tutor commented in the Mock Exam Report that I was always willing to help and to join in activities, that I was able to converse on a wide number of subjects and he was sure that in time I would overcome my difficulties. My subject tutors were also complimentary.

I felt that finally I was winning against the difficulties that my disabilities had caused me. I had cracked it – I was going to achieve academic success after all! But I knew that the real test was still to come – the CSEs themselves.

These exams took place in July. I was very nervous on the day of the first exam – I felt desperately worried to the point where I felt physically sick. Every ten minutes I needed to visit the loo – I was an emotional wreck!

Once the exams started, they steamed ahead. That first day I had one English paper in the morning and another in the afternoon. The next day I had to sit two Maths papers. I quickly became worn out – as I had feared, I was uncomfortable sitting down and the pain in my hands soon became unbearable.

The next exam was Art – and strangely my hands did not hurt at all, probably because I was no longer panicking, but relaxed and immersed in my artwork. For the exam I had to draw and paint two famous buildings in England. I chose Number Ten Downing Street (because ten was my favourite number) and the Houses of Parliament because that had always been my favourite building. I felt that the exam had gone well, and I was really happy afterwards.

By contrast, I did not even take the Biology exam. I did not want to put myself through any more trauma – and I told myself that anyway I did not need a qualification in that subject. I was determined by now to study Art – I knew that I would need Maths and English to get into college, but decided Biology was totally unnecessary.

My exams played on my mind in the following days. I had a nasty feeling that I had failed English and Maths, and this worried me. My mother arranged a meeting with Mr Cotton, and I told him about my worries.

'Don't give it another thought,' he said. 'It really doesn't matter. I have a plan for you anyway. What do you think about doing an extra year at Twynham? We could bring you up to scratch with the English and Maths, to prepare you for college. Your teacher tells me you want to become an artist'.

I wasn't sure how I felt about staying at school, studying with the children in the year below me. The headteacher was kind and understood my hesitation. He told me that I could have a couple of weeks to think about it.

Soon after the exams were over I started to play football with my friends on Farmer Bailey's field again. I was always the goalie – I found this better than playing mid-field as I was still participating in the game but had less chance of getting injured.

The holidays were over soon. I had failed my exams as I had expected, and I took Mr Cotton up on his offer and went back to Twynham for an extra year. To encourage me, he put me in top groups and made me study not just English and Maths, but also History, General Science, Biology and Art. Because I was only studying six subjects I had plenty of free time between lessons, which were filled with extra art classes.

I was seventeen that year. I just stayed in my pyjamas the whole day and watched television – I had decided not to have a party that year but felt that I should mark the occasion of my birthday somehow!

I was given a new bike, which had been built especially for me by a friend's father. I sold my old spider bike to the boy who lived next door, although I knew I would miss it. My new bike had a specially lowered saddle and shortened pedals, and I rode it for years, all over town and out to the Forest.

At school I was taking General Science, and I did a special project on Concorde. The others in my class did not have projects – but then I had come into a new year group in the middle of their exam studies, so the work set for me was slightly different.

I enjoyed the Concorde project, and learned a lot. English lessons were a struggle though – I had to study

Shakespeare, which was new to me. I was told to read from 'Romeo and Juliet' to the class. I acted out the parts as I read them, and did very well, but when I was asked to write an essay about the play I had no idea where to start. Shakespeare was simply not my cup of tea.

Maths was like Double Dutch to me. I had never been in the top group before, and I had no idea at all about algebra. I cringed inwardly when I heard my name called. 'What does Pi mean?' the teacher asked.

'Well, it doesn't mean anything, Sir,' I said, 'You are supposed to put it in the oven, and eat it'.

Everybody burst out laughing, which pleased me – I would rather have my classmates laugh with me than at me. Anyway, when would I ever need to know about Pi in my ordinary life? As long as I could add up and take away, that was fine. I didn't see why I should by tormented by algebra.

Biology lessons were far more enjoyable. I liked learning about the human body, and understood it well. One day the teacher asked me to talk to the rest of the class about my operation, and I agreed.

'Boys and girls,' she said. 'Can you name the bone that Antony had taken away from his knee, during the very serious operation that he had at Great Ormond Street Hospital?'

'Is it the patella, Miss?' asked a girl.

'No, but that's close,' replied the teacher.

Nobody knew, so the teacher asked me to tell the class. I explained that it was the femur bone. 'It had overgrown,' I told them. 'It looked like two tennis balls, and was very painful'.

I decided to give the class a talk about my structure and how Morquio's Syndrome, a genetic disorder, had caused my problems. I told them how I was better now, because I had stopped growing and so the effects of Morquio's had retreated. The teacher was really pleased that I had spoken about it, and thanked me effusively before I sat down, saying that it had taught the class a great deal.

Art was still my favourite subject of course, and my teachers put every effort into helping me to produce an impressive portfolio.

Life was not all school work – I had hobbies too. I still loved music, and I had built up quite a collection of vinyl records. I enjoyed all sorts of music, including classic, film soundtrack, and pop.

One day a friend of my Uncle Matt gave me a present of a big box full of vinyl records. There were two British bands in there which I particularly liked – a Supertramp album which featured the hit Dreamer, and a Uriah Heep album called Salisbury, which had a picture of a tank on the front cover.

I was so pleased with my growing collection that I catalogued it painstakingly, using my old ribboned typewriter. When my Mum and Dad went out I used to turn up the volume on the music centre as loud as it would go and blast out the sounds... It was bliss.

I was also interested in fashion. Most of the boys at school wore flared trousers and platform shoes at that time. Mum had to make me some flared trousers to fit, because I was only 4ft 9. However, I was ahead of the times – I had been wearing platform shoes for sometime already, or at least one of them (the built up shoe on my right foot!). I grew my hair long, to fit in with my general image. I looked very cool and with it!

Then my friends and I moved over to a new look, which included tie-dye T-shirts and funny-shaped tinted sunglasses. We would chew gum, wear cool waistcoats and generally look, or at least feel, groovy.

I remember 1976 as the year when I heard Demis Roussos singing Forever and Ever for the first time. I had gone into a second hand shop in Purewell and heard wonderful music playing in the background. I asked the shopkeeper who was singing and when he told me I rushed up to my local record shop to buy my first Demis Roussos album. It cost me £3.85 and it was worth every penny.

In February I took mock exams in English, Maths, History, Art, General Science and Biology. I passed some, but not all of the subjects. And of course, I did well in Art – and was delighted to be told that I would be taking the O' level in May. O' (for 'Ordinary') was a higher level exam than CSE, and it was an honour to be entered for an O' level – it meant that your teachers thought you would do better than average.

My House Tutor and House Master commented on my Mock Exam Report, saying that I made great efforts with all my work, and had a very good attitude towards my studies. Mr Cotton added some encouraging words too – he said that, 'Antony's cheerful application is an example and tonic to everyone' which I thought was a nice thing to say. I got on well with Mr Cotton – I felt that he understood me.

The 'real' exams took place in the main school hall. The pressure was on – I felt that a lot depended on these results. I had prepared as well as I could, even teaching myself to write with both hands in case the pain became too much for my right hand!

I actually found the CSE exams quite easy. However, my hands did hurt from trying to write so much, so fast, and this held me back. Also, my hips were causing me intense pain from having to sit in one position for so long. I tried to pull myself together, and did somehow manage to answer the questions, although I was not sure that I had done so to the best of my ability.

My Art O' level exam took place in the art studio. I had to draw a building which included many tower blocks, and paint it in watercolour, with small paintbrushes. I was quite happy with my work, but knew I would have to wait several months to find out how I had done.

Not long after the exams I had an interview with Mr Ted Tudgay and Mr Michael Goth at the Bournemouth and Poole College of Art. This was then located in the Royal London House in Lansdowne Road in Bournemouth.

I showed them my art portfolio, and they were very impressed with my plumbing designs – pictures of pipes, ballcocks and so on, inspired by my Dad's work – and my designs of buildings. Mr Goth asked whether I thought I could cope with a three year course, bearing in mind my disability. I said that I would certainly do my best.

The two of them kept looking at my work and conferring between themselves in low voices. Eventually I became impatient and burst out, 'Well, what do you think?' They then asked me to wait outside while they made a decision. When they called me back in again, Mr Tudgay said, 'Congratulations. You have been accepted to do a one year foundation course and then a two year Graphic Design and History of Art Diploma course at Royal London House. You will start at the end of September this year'.

I was delighted to hear this, and thanked them effusively. I left Royal London House feeling as though I was walking on air, and the next day at school I went straight to find my art teachers, Mr Phillips and Mrs Shave, to share the good news with them. The pair of them literally cried with joy, and Mrs Shave gave me a big hug, telling me that I had done amazingly well to fight my way right up to the top and win a place at college. I was so pleased to have made them both so proud – by now I felt that they had become my friends as well as my teachers.

The next day was my very last day at Twynham School. I was sad about this. I went to see Mr Cotton in his office for one last time. 'Congratulations, Antony, about your place at college,' he told me. 'And by the way, I want to talk to you about something. You see, I have figured out your secret'.

I said nothing, just looked at him and waited.

'I have realised,' said my headteacher, 'That you have

great talent. If you had not been disabled I am convinced that you would have been in the top classes right throughout your time at this school. It was your disability that held you back – causing you problems and preventing you from achieving your full potential. Am I right, Antony?'

'You are, Sir,' I said, 'You have guessed my secret. I didn't want to bring attention to my disability, because I thought I might be moved to another school, one for disabled children. And I love being at Twynham – I always have!'

'You needn't have worried about that,' said Mr Cotton. 'There would always have been a place for you here. But I am very impressed with your strength of mind and determination. I would like to give you a small gift on behalf of the school. We have all benefited from having you here, and we will never forget you. Well done, son'.

The gift was a digital watch with a calculator and I loved it – I wore it for many years afterwards. I loved it most for what it symbolised – that I was special, because no other pupil who left Twynham had ever been given a gift before.

Mr Cotton then invited all my other tutors into his office to say goodbye. I felt truly honoured, but also sad – it was so hard to leave that school, where I had known such happy times.

It was the summer holidays now, and I had no plans. I just took things easy, and waited for my exam results. When they arrived I was disappointed to find out that I had failed my English and Biology CSEs. I had passed my Art O'level though, with a grade B, which I was over the moon about. And I had my place at the Bournemouth and Poole College of Art to look forward to, which was fantastic.

Chapter Seventeen
College

I started my new course in September. I enjoyed the course, made friends and got on well with the tutors. I did not like the building we studied in though. Ascham House was very old and run down, dark and dusty. It was a bit spooky too – there were mirrors everywhere. There was no lift, but luckily I could manage the stairs, which were wide and shallow.

I generally did very well at the Foundation course, and enjoyed my studies – except for the life drawing classes. I was embarrassed by having to draw naked models, and particularly taken aback when our first model turned out to be a middle aged lady. For the class, all of the students were assembled in front of our easels in the main hall, and the lady was on a small stage in front of us.

She was totally starkers, but she looked nothing like I had ever seen in the adult magazines my friends bought – her boobs were hanging down as though she had somehow got a slow puncture in them. The poor lady was doing her best to pose naturally without moving in front of our group of young college students. After a while though, she could not hold her pose any longer, so she shifted uncomfortably - and suddenly the stage gave way. The lady's weight brought it tumbling down with a mighty crash.

I could not stop laughing, from embarrassment and relief. The best thing was that the life class was then postponed to another day. I never saw that poor naked lady again.

We then moved on to a short photography course. I found this great fun. I was quite fit in those days, and it was no effort at all to spend the day walking around Bournemouth taking photos. Developing the pictures gave me awful headaches though, because of the chemicals. I also found the lack of daylight in the darkroom disorientating, and got confused about whether it was night or day when it was time to head home. I persevered though, and became quite handy with a camera.

We had to do other projects, including making scale models and creating advertising posters. I made a poster of the glamorous Swedish tennis player, Bjorn Borg. I found him quite inspirational, and I even took to copying his style, wearing a headband around my hair, which was really long by then. I was proud of my work, and disappointed when I handed it in to my tutors for marking and never saw it again.

1977 was the year of the Queen's Silver Jubilee. I went on a special trip with my sister Julie and my Uncle Matt to see a review of the Royal Navy fleet at Spithead. We sailed to the Solent and toured around the Royal Navy ships there, along with hundreds of other people who had also paid for the privilege.

There were so many different boats on display – it was a very impressive occasion. To crown it all, there was the Queen's yacht, the Royal Yacht Britannia. I squinted hard, and made out the Queen herself on deck – everybody on our boat gave a spontaneous cheer!

I did feel a little uncomfortable though – I was suffering from seasickness. A passing waiter noticed and he advised me to 'dance with the boat' – swaying in an opposite direction to the flow of the waves. To my surprise, this worked well.

Evening came, and enhanced our experience – now we could see the HMS ships lit up against the night sky. They were all anchored side by side, and looked fantastic, like floating ghost ships in the dark. I was so grateful to Matt for bringing Julie and I to see this wonderful sight.

The excitement was not over yet. Around that time all our neighbours gathered together to arrange a street party to celebrate the Silver Jubilee. I hosted the party and organised all the music.

A lot of organisation went into that street party. Several days before, my friends and I had started collecting wood for the Jubilee bonfire. On the day of the party itself, we bedecked the whole street in bunting and balloons. A great long table (made up of lots of smaller ones) was placed in the middle of the street, with dozens of chairs around it.

Everybody pitched in, all contributing food. No detail went unattended to – the tables were decorated and laid with paper plates and cups, and everybody wore party clothes and party hats. And the festivities did not end with the meal – they went on long into the evening, with pony rides (ponies supplied from Ashtree House courtesy of Uncle Matt) a wheel barrow race, sack race, egg and spoon race, and of course plenty of dancing and drinking.

It was soon July, and my first year at college was drawing to a close. I was studying history of art now, and I enjoyed this. I liked the work of the Renaissance artists, particularly Michaelangelo and Raphael, and learning about their lives was fascinating.

When the summer holidays arrived I was surprised to learn that the college would be closed for ten whole weeks. I had assumed that we would have six weeks off, as we had always done at school. Ten weeks was too long to be inactive, so I got a job washing up at a local hotel. It was exhausting work, and I soon switched to another hotel, where I worked in the evenings from seven o'clock until midnight, earning seventy-five pence each hour. I liked that job, because the family who ran the place were very kind to me and very generous – on occasions they would let my whole family enjoy an evening meal at the hotel, free of charge.

One day I went fly fishing with my Grandad. He had asked me to take him to Claypool to fish, because I was a member of Christchurch Angling Club. 'I'll take you,' I said, 'But you won't catch a thing'.

'You'll see,' Grandad said as we walked down the bank, past the other fishermen and the boats. 'I'm going to show you how to catch a big fish'.

To my surprise, Grandad did not put his bait (a fly) directly on the line, but wrapped it in the silver wrapper of a Kit-Kat first. 'Why are you doing that?' I asked.

'Shh,' he said. 'Be quiet and you'll learn something'.

I was impressed when Grandad landed a big fish. However, the bailiff was right behind him when the fish was on the line. Grandad hesitated to pull it out of the water, and by the time he did reel the line in, the fish had gone. I realised that he hadn't wanted the bailiff to see the silver paper – because it was against the Club rules to fish in this way. The bailiff knew what Grandad was up to, but hadn't caught him at it, so there was nothing he could do. Foiled again!

'Why do you have to cheat, Grandad?' I asked.

'I'm not cheating!' he insisted. I suppose he meant that in his opinion the rules did not apply to him.

I worked throughout those summer holidays, and I saved every penny that I earned. With my wages I bought a Sanyo Stereo music centre, which sounded wonderful and had all sorts of knobs and buttons – volume, bass, treble, FM, long wave and medium wave radio, a tape recorder with two stereo microphones and a record deck with two speakers. It cost £220 – an absolute fortune, and it left me completely skint, but I never regretted buying it for a minute. It was my pride and joy!

Now I had to find a way to get music to play on my centre. I was very crafty – instead of buying records I listened to them on the radio and recorded them onto a blank cassette tape. So I was cheating too, in a way, but like Grandad I decided that those particular rules did not apply to me. And I was generous with my skill – I recorded a lot of free music for my friends too!

Back at college in September I embarked on a special two year foundation course. I took Graphic Design and Commercial Advertising and Marketing (quite a mouthful!). I was studying in Royal London House now, not Ascham House, and I liked this building much better. It was in the centre of Lansdowne, right among the banks and businesses.

It was a very busy spot, and there was a good bus service. It was all very noisy and crowded, outside the college and within it. I felt overwhelmed at first by all the noise and bustle, and often felt hemmed in and at risk of being squashed by the crowds. I had to push my way through the other students to get to my classes on time, and I felt intimidated by this, because I was smaller than the others. I was lucky though, to be able to use the lift – because my classes were on the fifth floor and I might have become quite tired otherwise!

The art studio had a great view, looking down onto the busy roundabout outside, and all the shops. Right below Royal London House was a well known coffee shop, Fortes, and although it was expensive, we students would sometimes treat ourselves to a drink or a snack there. It's all gone down market now unfortunately – Fortes has been replaced by a Kentucky Fried Chicken outlet!

I caught a Bournemouth Yellow Bus each morning, from my home in Purewell to the College. It took about twenty minutes, and I usually didn't mind the journey. One day though, I started to cough and couldn't stop – and I noticed that all of the other passengers were coughing too. The driver said the problem was caused by battery fumes from the engine and advised us all to drink milk when we arrived at our destination, to counteract the effect of the fumes. Luckily this strategy worked, and we did not find ourselves in this dangerous position again.

I enjoyed the routine of college. Each lunchtime I walked to Wilkins the bakers - I was addicted to their long cheese rolls and thin fried chips. The manager of the shop was really kind to me – he used to get my lunch ready every day before I arrived. When I came in to collect it he would call out, 'Let this young disabled man through please,' and I would go to the head of the long queue to collect my lunch.

One of my college friends used to tell me off for eating so many chips. He said they were made from dried potato powder, like 'Smash' the instant mash, and that it would turn me into an alien (the 'Smash' adverts featured aliens). I knew he was right, not about me turning into an alien, but that the chips had bad fats in them – but I liked them so much that I felt powerless to resist!

I was working late at college one evening when I got taken ill. The principal, Mr Tudgay, took me home in his car. I had been overworking and not eating well, and was light-headed and faint. I took several days to recover, and realised afterwards that I needed to take better care of myself, and listen to my body when it told me to rest.

I handed in another piece of coursework in October – I had designed a shop display – and I was disappointed again when my work was not returned to me after it had been graded. I complained, but I still never saw my work again. The same thing happened with a British Rail poster I designed, and I realised that it must be college policy to hold onto our work.

I was nineteen that year and I received a great present from my Mum and Dad – a Demis Rousoss album called 'Magic'. And magic it was too, with the big hit 'Because' which I loved.

In December, Star Wars was released. Everyone was very excited about this film, queuing outside the cinemas in freezing temperatures to buy tickets to see it. I wasn't particularly interested, but my friend persuaded me to go with him. I was not very impressed with the film, although I like it better now – it has grown on me!

I was coming up to the half-way mark of my three year college Art course, and the time seemed to have gone very fast. At the start of the January term I made a new friend, someone who became very special to me. I was working late at Royal London House one night, trying to finish off one of my illustrations. I looked at my watch, and was shocked to see that it was almost eight pm. I didn't want to miss the bus home, so I packed up hurriedly, shoving all my art materials and sketchbooks haphazardly into my briefcase.

I ran full pelt to the lift. However, it seemed to take an age to arrive (I was on the fifth floor) so I decided to go down the steps instead. I was only two steps away from the ground floor when I stumbled and fell, landing in a heap on the solid concrete floor.

I landed head down. All my art work and materials spilled from my briefcase as I fell. My nose was bleeding and my arm hurt terribly, but fortunately I was still conscious.

And that was when I saw Ellie for the first time. A girl, about my age, came down the stairs and saw me lying on the floor. She picked me up and made me sit on the nearby steps to recover. She sat next to me, holding my hand, and I couldn't help noticing that she was lovely looking, with long light brown hair, the front section plaited over her forehead.

Ellie insisted on driving me home. I had already noticed

that she was not English, although she spoke the language very well. In the car she told me that she was French and lived in Nice, but had come to England to study fashion design.

I told her that I was studying Graphic Design and History of Art. I directed Ellie to Ashtree House, and she was very impressed when we arrived at our destination. I explained that it was my Grandad's house – I was staying with Grandad because my Mum and Dad happened to be on holiday that week. What I didn't tell Ellie was that they didn't trust me to be at home alone, in case I invited my friends over for any wild parties!

I introduced Ellie to my Grandad and Nanny and we explained what had happened at college. Grandad thanked Ellie for her kind help, she left, and I staggered up to bed.

I was slow to get up the next morning – I ached from my fall, and was badly bruised. Suddenly Grandad called me, 'Time to get up Antony! Your breakfast is ready, and is getting cold. And your friend Ellie has arrived'.

Well that was an unexpected surprise – I had hoped to bump into Ellie again at college soon, but had no idea that she would turn up on my doorstep so soon! I hurried downstairs and into the sun lounge, where she was waiting.

'How are you feeling now?' she asked.

'Not great,' I told her.

Ellie kept me company while I had breakfast, and then

drove me into college. I arrived at Royal London House just in time for my History of Art lecture, and Ellie went off to her fashion design course. When my lecture had finished, I headed off to work in the library. I liked studying in there – there were huge tables to spread out on, and stacks of books in the tall shelves. The librarians were kind and friendly, and sometimes assisted me when I couldn't find or reach what I wanted.

Suddenly, Ellie turned up again! 'Ah, so this is where you've been hiding, Antony!' she exclaimed. 'Come on, I'm taking you out for lunch'.

Ellie and I quickly became firm friends. We ate lunch together every day, often in the fashion design studio where she worked on her embroidery. She was two years older than me, and very pretty – I was always proud to be seen with her. She designed wedding dresses, which were stunning works of art.

One day I asked Ellie why she'd come to England to study, when she would have been snapped up by any college in her native France.

'Ah, but I wanted to study in England,' she told me. 'I simply love English fashion and history. Especially anything to do with the royal family, or with Twiggy – sixties fashion was the best!'

'I like Twiggy too,' I said, 'And believe it or not, I like fashion. We seem to have so much in common, you and I. Is there anything else you want to tell me?'

We laughed – we always laughed so easily together. We found time to see each other often, although we still both put a lot of effort into our respective college courses. At the weekends we took trips in Ellie's Mini Cooper, often to the New Forest. We were becoming closer by the day.

I did not tell my Mum about Ellie, because I knew that she would worry about me getting hurt. One day Grandad asked me to go to Ashtree for 'a chat'. He had obviously been watching, because he brought up the subject of Ellie. He said that he was glad I had met a nice girl, and that he realised I was an adult now. But, he warned, 'Be careful. You could end up heartbroken'.

Grandad said that I should see other friends at the weekends, not just Ellie. He also said that I should take the bus to college and back, to maintain my independence (Ellie had fallen into the habit of giving me lifts to and from college each day). Nothing had been going on really, but I took his advice and after that Ellie and I were still close, but not as exclusive as we had been. I started to see my other friends again, and my social life branched out.

Chapter Eighteen
May Day!

In March of 1978, a memorable event occurred . I had just got home from college and Mum and Dad had gone out, but left my dinner in the oven.

I ate, then settled down to listen to music. I turned the dial on my radio slowly, wondering what to tune into. Suddenly I heard some morse code – dot, dot, dash... and then a voice, sharp and urgent, calling, 'May Day! May Day!'

I was shocked, and a little confused. I thought at first that it was a radio drama or documentary, but soon realised that was not the case. I rang my Grandad, who told me to call the police. So I did, reporting the morse code signal and the May Day call. I was assured that the police would alert the Coastguard.

I heard nothing for a while after that, so I left the house, and went over to visit my Grandad. Soon Mum and Dad arrived - they had been shopping and had picked up some provisions for Grandad too, and were dropping them off.

They were surprised to see me at Ashtree House, and I explained what had happened. Just then there was a firm knocking at the door.

A police officer stood there. He explained that a neighbour had sent him over from our house. I had given my name and address when I made my call to the police, and this officer had come to see me.

'You saved many lives tonight son,' the police officer

said. 'You were the only person who picked up that May Day call. Because of the speed and accuracy with which you reported it, we were able to locate the vessel in distress, which was a one thousand ton cargo vessel, the Lune Fisher, in the North Sea. The cargo had shifted, and the vessel was listing badly. I dread to think what the outcome might have been if you had not managed to alert the authorities, who came to their rescue'.

I was so happy and honoured to have helped those seamen. I couldn't believe that my action had saved their lives, and their cargo. I was so proud. I was interviewed by the Bournemouth Evening Echo, who featured a photograph of me with my music centre. I was also interviewed on Radio Solent. And following that was a longer Echo article, with more detail on the story.

I was hailed as a local hero. But as I told the interviewers, it was pure luck that I had been the right place at the right time. I explained how the signal had come across quite clearly, and I talked them through my stereo equipment and what it could do. Although I had no shipping band and just an ordinary domestic radio receiver, I could usually listen in to police, fire and ambulance calls on the VHF channel. (That was quite usual in those days – although now the police transmit on a different frequency, which is much better protected from the public.)

I was pleased when all the fuss had died down – although at the end of March I received a handwritten letter from the Captain of the Lune Fisher. He said that he wanted to thank me personally for helping to save his life and the lives of his crew members, and with the letter he enclosed a cheque for £50. I did not want to accept the money – I felt that I had only done what anybody would do in such circumstances and that I did not deserve a reward. I wrote to say so, but the captain insisted that I should keep the money – so I did, and I put it towards buying my next music centre.

After all the excitement, it was now time for the Easter break from art college. Ellie went back to France to spend time with her parents, and I took the opportunity to catch up with my other friends.

Easter Sunday morning brought a good crop for me – I had five large chocolate eggs from family and friends. Mum told me not to have too much chocolate, because there would be a big roast dinner to tuck into later. I was hungry though, and so I started nibbling away. It was so delicious that one bite led to another, and before I realised what I had done, I had demolished all five eggs!

I felt very full, and slightly panicky. Mum called me for lunch, and I walked very slowly to the kitchen. I was not happy to see the huge plate of food that she set down in front of me. She looked at me suspiciously. 'Have you been at those Easter eggs, Antony?' she asked. 'I hope you are going to eat your dinner now, because otherwise there will be trouble'.

I managed to put some food on my fork and tentatively raised it to my mouth. But then – horror of horrors – I had to dash immediately to the toilet, where I was very sick indeed. Mum said I went as white as a sheet! I had to admit that she had been right as usual – I should not have eaten so much chocolate in the morning! It took me several days to recover, and I swore that I would never eat chocolate again.

Later in the holidays, Uncle Matt invited me to Grandad's house to play snooker. I was on a winning streak that day and Matt was not a gracious loser. He moaned and groaned, and eventually gave in.

'Why don't you invite your friend Garry to play with you instead?' he suggested.

Garry and I spent most evenings playing snooker after that. One day he suggested that we play the best out of three matches, and that the winner would get a bar of chocolate.

'Oh help, not chocolate,' I thought to myself. 'I don't like the sound of that' and I deliberately let him win the games! (I must admit that I have weakened since then – I broke my vow never to eat chocolate again and now I indulge occasionally, especially in Swiss chocolate. But I have never eaten so much chocolate as to make myself sick since that fateful Easter day!)

The holidays were over by the middle of April, and I was glad to get back to college and see Ellie again. I had missed her. She asked whether I'd had plenty of chocolate eggs for Easter and so I told her the story of what had happened and how I'd made myself sick by over-indulging.

'You should stick to your two finger Kit-Kats,' she said, which made me smile, because I hadn't realised that she had noticed my predilection for those particular chocolate bars. 'You are a Cadbury's fruit and nut case,' I told her, and for some reason we both got the giggles, like children sharing a joke that only they can understand.

Ellie kissed me on the cheek then. 'Meet me at half past twelve for lunch,' she said. 'Outside the Round House Hotel'. We went our separate ways for the morning then – and my art tutor gave me the brief for my next project, which was to design an illustration for the cover of the Sunday Times magazine. The illustration would be for an article on the effects of the Japanese motor industry on British Leyland's market. Cheap and well-made Japanese cars were now flooding into Britain, as motorbikes had done during my last years at Twynham, and our tutors thought that to illustrate an article on this subject would make an interesting brief for us.

Anyway, later on I went to meet Ellie outside the Round House Hotel, which was just opposite Royal London House. Suddenly a pair of hands covered my eyes, and a voice called out, 'Guess who?!'

'Hi Ellie,' I said. 'Why are we eating here? It's so expensive'.

'Don't worry,' she told me. 'I'm paying. Actually, I'm staying in this hotel now. I wasn't happy in my digs, and my father has paid for me to stay here until my course finishes'.

We both had the afternoon off college, so after a lovely lunch we went down to the nearby beach at Bournemouth. It was a very warm day for the time of year, and we sat on the sand for ages, talking about ourselves and our families. It was clear to me that our relationship was progressing to another level.

'Can I ask you something, Ellie?' I said.

'You're going to ask whether I have a boyfriend,' she

said. 'The answer is, no'.

I felt so nervous and emotional, and to my embarrassment I began to cry. I told her that I had never had a girlfriend before. 'Well, you have one now,' she said. 'You have me'.

We were both crying now. 'I don't want you to think I am using you,' she said. 'I don't care what you look like, that you're short and have to wear special shoes. I just think you're kind and funny, and I like you'.

So Ellie and I were now officially a couple. But we were both clear that we should act like adults, and balance our friendship and college work. I hadn't forgotten my promise to my Grandad – even though I was really pleased to have a girlfriend at last!

I got stuck into my latest art project at college now. I went to the Russell Cotes Art Gallery in Bournemouth town centre for inspiration. I read lots of books on mythology. I even interviewed a garage proprietor, who sold Japanese cars. I put a lot of effort and imagination into this work, and came up with a design that I was proud of – a Japanese Samurai warrior chasing a tyre (which symbolised British Leyland) down a slope.

I handed the work in, and again I was disappointed when it was never returned to me. I wondered what on earth was happening to all my work, and although I did not want to rock the boat at college, I resolved that I would confront my tutors about the matter at some point.

I was busy these days, but when I was at home I still liked to watch the television. British television was starting to show more American dramas. My favourites included Chips, Mork and Mindy, Happy Days, Charlie's Angels and Starsky and Hutch.

The first time I saw the American TV comedy Taxi I was amazed. The star was a small man called Danny DeVito – at four feet nine inches he was exactly the same height as me! I found the show really funny, and DeVito made me happy at a deeper level – seeing him so comfortable in his own skin made me feel better, and gave me the courage to face up to taller people in the streets, without feeling inadequate. It just did me the world of good psychologically, to have that role model on the television.

It was the World Cup again this year, from the 1st to the 25th June. The Cup was hosted by Argentina. I was biting my nails, hoping that my beautiful team Brazil would win. I watched each and every game in the series, and could even tell you today which game was won by which country, and by how many goals! However, the upshot of it all was not good news for me – Argentina won the cup, Holland came second and Brazil was just third place.

It was the summer holidays now, and my hair had grown so long and thick that I was starting to look and feel like a Yetti. I went to a local hairdresser's to have it layered and styled. It was still long, but more manageable now. The holidays went by fast – I did small jobs at Ashtree Riding School to earn extra money.

In September I returned to college to start my final year of studies. Ellie and I were very close by now, and managed to spend a lot of time together, although both of us had a lot of college work to do.

In November I saw my first Demis Roussos concert, at the Winter Gardens in Bournemouth. Unfortunately Ellie could not accompany me as she had a bad case of flu. My friend came along though, and at my request he fixed my small tape recorder onto his leg, and so managed to record the concert! Fortunately for both of us, he did not get caught.

Christmas played out according to the usual routine - lunch cooked by Mum at home and then my Grandad's Christmas tea party at Ashtree House. 1979 was upon us now, and already I was dreading the parting that I knew was ahead – because, of course, Ellie was due to return to her home country when she graduated from college, and I knew that I would miss her dreadfully when she left.

I went back to college knowing that I just had a few months left of my course. The original plan was to progress onto the Diploma course, but I no longer wanted to do this. I felt that I was ready now to take what I had learned out into the world and use it in the workplace.

I met the Principal of the College, Mr Tudgay, in his office. He told me that he was very pleased with my creative designs. 'Have you anything you wish to discuss with me, Antony?' he asked.

'Well, yes actually,' I said. 'I have really enjoyed the last few years at college, and feel that I have benefited from my studies, and from socialising with the other students.'. I then explained that I did not want to continue onto the Diploma.

Mr Tudgay said that this was fine, and that although I would not be entitled to a certificate to show that I had achieved a qualification, my years of hard work should count for something. He said that he would put his mind to finding a solution.

Meanwhile, I started a new project. It was called 'Skin Deep' and the idea was to design an advert for ladies' cosmetics. I put a lot of time and thought into this, and came up with a pleasing design, comprising various images of make-up in progress, and a fully made-up face at the end (I took a photo of a friend to illustrate this).

Around that time, Ellie and I had a day out together. She was interested in my home town of Christchurch and she suggested that we tour the area together. I protested that it sounded too tiring, but she insisted, 'Come on, it'll be fun. I'll hold you up if you get worn out, or we'll find a seat for you to rest on.'

So I gave in. We bought a tour guide booklet in Roberts Toys and Gifts Shop, and plodded around Christchurch, visiting the Priory, Christchurch Quay, the Old Mill, the Red House Museum, the Ducking Stool, the castle ruins and Constable House. Then we went to the Copper Skillet, where we ate gammon and chips, followed by an ice-cream sundae. My legs were hurting now, so Ellie drove me back to Ashtree House, where we had a cup of tea with Grandad. It had been a great day out.

I saw Ellie a lot during the Easter holidays – she did not return to France this year. She always called me Anton instead of Antony, and one day I asked her why.

'It is more romantic,' she replied. It sounds cool. And it suits you better. You should call yourself Anton'.

I could see that she was sincere, and I liked the name. So gradually I switched (although not by deed poll) and nowadays all my friends and family know me as Anton. It was hard for my Mum and Dad to remember at first, but now my Mum even signs our family Christmas cards 'from June, Jim and Anton'.

On Easter Sunday one of my friends asked me to accompany him to church, so I agreed. I fell asleep during the long service, and only woke up when the congregation was singing the final hymn. 'Oh Jesus, I have promised to serve you to the end,' it went, but as I joined in I changed the words, 'Oh Jesus I have promised to stay awake to the end..' I was trying to make my friend laugh. I also pulled my old trick of pretending to put a donation into the collection box, but palming the money instead. I was not the best of churchgoers!

In May, I voted for the first time in my life, at the polling station in Somerford. Uncle Matt took me, and kept pestering me to tell him who I voted for. ' The Monster Raving Loonies,' I said, 'Because they have more sense than all the others put together'.

The Tories got in, of course, with Margaret Thatcher making history as the first ever female Prime Minister in this country. I am not saying who I really voted for – but I will say that it wasn't the Raving Loonies!

I was now really coming close to the end of my time at the Bournemouth and Poole College of Art. The principal came up trumps, arranging a special reference for me, which said that I worked with consistent industry, that I was well-liked, punctual and polite and completely honest and that I would be a reliable and cheerful employee.

With this letter, I felt sure that I would soon get a good job. I left Mr Tudgay's office in a very good mood, but then I got the most horrendous shock.

Ellie's friend was waiting for me in the library. She said that my girlfriend was seriously ill, that she had gone back to France, and would contact me when possible. Although Ellie's friend was very kind, I was devastated. I had no address for my girlfriend in France, and so I could not check on her health until she called me. I gave Ellie's friend my phone number, so that she could pass on any news, and went about my business sadly.

It was time to give back all my books, and to say goodbye to my friends and tutors. I did all of it with a heavy heart, because all I could think of was Ellie, and what on earth could be wrong with her.

The day was over, and it was time to catch the bus home from college for the last time. I did one last thing before I left – I crossed the busy road to stand on the Lansdowne roundabout. I could see the college, as well as all the surrounding shops and businesses.

'Thank you Royal London House,' I said, looking over at the building. An awful lot had happened to me during my time there – I had grown up, learned a lot, met Ellie... I had a lump in my throat just thinking about it. Sadly I crossed back over, and stood waiting for the bus to carry me home, where the next phase of my life would begin.

I had a difficult few weeks, waiting for news from Ellie.

Finally she called – a very quick, sad phone call, just to say goodbye. She told me she'd been very ill, although she didn't specify what was wrong. She said that she was sorry that we hadn't been able to say goodbye properly.

I told her not to worry. I also assured her that I would go by the name of Anton from now on, because it would make me feel as if she was part of me forever. 'Goodbye, Anton,' she said finally. 'I love you'.

'I love you too', I said. 'I love you so much, Ellie'. And then the phone crackled and the call ended – my French Connection was broken, and I felt as though my heart was breaking too.

Chapter Nineteen
Searching for Work

We held my 21st birthday party at St Joseph's church hall, in Purewell. It was a fancy dress party – I dressed as my hero, Demis Roussos. Mum helped me with the costume – she put pillows around me for padding, and I wore a long kaftan. Dad provided some hemp from his plumbing work, which we dyed and made into a wig. Everybody had great fun, and I knew that it was an occasion which I would remember.

In November my cousin asked whether I would help to design and build a big pirate ship for a carnival float. It looked brilliant when it was finished – a proper old-style galleon, with tall sails, and we won the Rose Bowl Trophy (the top prize in the carnival).

In the New Year of 1980 I decided to take an adult education course. It turned out that Mr Phillips, who had taught me art at school, was the tutor for the course. We studied for six months, every Wednesday evening for two hours, and I never missed a lesson.

Meanwhile, I was trying hard to find a job. The trouble was, companies would refuse me employment on the grounds that I had no work experience, which was a hard problem to fix. Another problem was that most companies had no facilities to employ disabled people, so that even if they wanted to give me a job they couldn't.

I found it dispiriting and disheartening to be out of work, and as time went on I felt myself crumbling under the pressure. Most people I knew defined themselves by the work they did and by their social activities, and to have no occupation and no money to spend made me feel very low indeed.

I spent day after day writing to various companies asking whether they had vacancies for a junior graphic artist. I spent a fortune on stamps - £42 – without getting one reply! I was close to giving up, when a friend told me that it would be better to send a stamped addressed envelope with my job enquiries. His advice worked to some extent - at least then I started to receive some rejection letters!

But each time another rejection letter arrived I was deeply disappointed. I knew I was not alone though – there were thousands of others out of work too. In fact, the UK was heading into a deep recession.

Grandad came to the rescue, sorting out a small evening job for me. He had a friend who was a jazz singer and who played the saxophone, and I was to help this friend to index his vinyl record collection. I was astounded the first time I went to the man's house – he had four thousand LPs that he wanted my help to catalogue! I was paid fifty pence an hour and I am afraid to say that I found the work so tedious that I only lasted a week there.

One afternoon my Uncle Matt called, and asked whether I would like to go to the cinema in Bournemouth with him – but I was feeling unwell, and said no. The next morning Matt came to our house in a state of high excitement. 'I have some incredible news, Anton!' he exclaimed. 'I saw an advert at the cinema last night, and they had used your design of Japanese Samurais, to illustrate the invasion of the British car industry. It was exactly like the idea you had at college'.

I had eventually received my work back from the college, and Matt had seen the picture in my portfolio. I was shocked and disappointed to hear that it had been used commercially without my knowledge or consent and my parents were furious. However, I reasoned that at least my work had reached a large audience. I still have the original design to this day.

I still had no success in finding work. Mum and Dad paid for my keep, and Grandad gave me some jobs at Ashtree House to earn some spending money. But I started to feel quite aimless and hopeless. I was falling into a deep depression, probably caused by the contrast between my years at college when I was busy, active, and challenged and my current situation of unemployment and inertia.

I was also feeling guilty, wondering whether I had contributed to my own downfall by deciding to be an artist instead of aiming for something that might have been easier to achieve. My Grandad reassured me on this point, reminding me that I was not the only one out of work in the UK – there were more than one and a half million of us!

One day I bumped into Ellie's friend from college, and we had a long chat. She told me that she had not managed to get a job either and was feeling very low, just like me. She'd had several interviews with fashion design companies, and she said that one job she'd applied for had over five hundred applicants!

Soon after that I had to go to Southampton General Hospital to see Mr Wilkinson about my bad hips. He X-rayed me and said that I had severe arthritis, and that quick action was needed before it got even worse.

'Will I need an operation?' I asked.

'Well, it is extremely serious,' he replied. 'The arthritis has grown inside your hip joint sockets and is affecting your balance quite badly. But I don't want to operate, and I don't believe it will be necessary. The best and most simple solution is for you to use an exercise bike to grind the arthritis away'.

'Also,' he went on, 'You should look into making a claim for Mobility Allowance.'

'What's that?' I asked.

'It is a grant from the Department of Health and Social Security,' he told me, 'You can get financial help to get you out and about. You could qualify for a Motability car'.

The next day, Mum and Dad bought a Puch exercise bike, adapted for my leg length. It had a timer and a tension lever – I had to work harder against the tension as I increased the settings. I used it daily, because I was determined to stay mobile.

In May I went for a medical examination to see whether I qualified for Mobility Allowance. I had two medicals actually - I failed the first medical deliberately, because I was convinced that if I qualified I would have to drive a three wheeler 'pop' car, which I thought was the most embarrassing vehicle I had ever seen!

It was only later that I realised I could have just taken the mobility allowance money, and used it for taxis or other forms of transport. So I had a second medical test, and was told I would have to wait until July for the results. I thought I had failed the test again, because the specialist who did the examination seemed very strict and stern.

In July I took my History of Art A level. It was not an easy exam, but I did my best. On the day the results arrived I was so nervous that I asked my Mum to open the envelope for me.

'You have done really well,' she said. 'You have not passed the A level, but you were so close that you got a Grade C 'O' level instead! That is a really good result – well done, son!'

Mum and Dad held a small party for me to celebrate. I looked at myself in the mirror that evening, and said to myself, 'One day, Anton, you will become a professional artist'. I really dared to hope it might be true!

More good news had come through the post – I had been awarded Mobility Allowance. Now I could get out and about a lot more, which cheered me up a lot. In September I embarked on a new project, studying fashion design at home.

Around the same time a friend asked me to help him design a piece of furniture. We came up with a design for a breakfast cabinet, which we managed to sell to a company in London, although we didn't get paid much for it.

My grandmother – Nanny Cook - died towards the end of that year. She had been poorly for some time, but we were still not prepared for her passing. She was a good grandmother, and I knew I would miss her – she had always looked after her grandchildren well, taking us on day trips out, often stopping at various cafes. She had played an active part at Ashtree Riding School too – she often catered for people on riding holidays, who stayed in Ashtree House.

At home, my Mum and Dad were both working hard to make ends meet. My Dad was suffering from angina, and although he still worked as a plumber he had to have regular hospital check ups, and take tablets to control his condition.

Dad had to cut back on work, and change his lifestyle. My Mum looked after him, and all of us, as she always had done. She was an educated person, and also very disciplined. Mum was healthy and strong in both body and mind, and she kept all of us on the straight and narrow. I used to call her HMS Battle Axe as she would never give in on any matter!

I remember doing a lot of jigsaw puzzles at that time. I spent two whole weeks watching the Snooker Championships, and I enjoyed every minute of every game, scoffing biscuits and slurping bucket loads of tea as I watched the action unfold on the screen.

I was demoralised because of my failure to get a job, and this began to affect my behaviour. Soon I refused to leave the house or make any effort to find something to do. I stayed in bed until lunchtime each day. I really was becoming bone idle.

My behaviour was abysmal – I did not care about anybody's feelings and I would be openly rude. My Mum and Dad were very concerned, although they understood that the reason I behaved like this was because I felt so hopeless about being out of work.

Mum tried to get me to go out to visit my friends or join a club, but I refused. I was still writing letters to companies asking for work, but the only replies I had said that they had no facilities to employ disabled people and I had no choice but to accept this.

One day I had a huge argument with my parents, railing at them and blaming them for my inability to get a job. I told my parents it was their fault that I could not find work, because they had caused me to be born disabled. I knew really that I was lucky that they continued to support me, but I hated feeling beholden to them.

My parents never blamed me, or made me feel bad about any of this, and Mum assured me that she was more than happy to pay for me to go out. I suppose it was better than having to put up with me staying indoors feeling sorry for myself! However, despite the understanding and support of my parents I sensed that I was becoming deeply depressed.

I could not sleep well at night, and had trouble relaxing in the daytimes. I seemed to be continually tense and anxious. I was bored and worried about my future, and these feelings manifested as aggression. I didn't see any friends socially, and if I was invited anywhere I made excuses, and didn't go.

I was frightened that I was on the verge of a breakdown. Some days I wanted to run away, but deep down I knew that was not the answer to my problems. I gradually declined, until the anxiety became full blown panic attacks. Mum stepped in to help, giving me a brown paper bag. She said I should hold it over my nose and mouth and breathe slowly in and out until I returned to normal. To my surprise this helped, and after that I took a paper bag with me whenever I went out – it was my 'First Aid Friend'!

I kept going somehow, working through the depression with the encouragement of my parents. Thank goodness for the wedding of Prince Charles and Lady Diana that summer, which seemed to lift everybody's mood. I was delighted when Princess Diana became the President of the Great Ormond Street Hospital for Sick Children.

I redoubled my efforts to find work, writing to all the companies I could think of, asking for a position as an apprentice Graphic Designer. I still had no luck – although the tone of the rejection letters had changed, and rather than saying they had no facilities to employ disabled people they now said that they only wanted people with prior work experience. This was immensely frustrating – how could I get work experience if nobody would give me a job?

One day, Uncle Matt asked whether I would like to accompany him to a goat farm in Lymington, about ten miles away. 'What do you want to go to a goat farm for?' I asked.

'I want to buy some goats to tidy up Ashtree,' he told me. 'They'll eat all the stinging nettles in the car park'.

When we arrived at the goat farm I was surprised by the scale of it – there were many hundreds of goats there, in an open barn, and they made an enormous racket. The owner showed us both around the farm, and asked me whether I would like to feed a baby goat, which I did, using a bottle.

'You really are good at that,' the farmer said. 'Would you like a weekend job?'

Matt said that he would sort out transport for me, and so I was pleased to accept. I started at the goat farm the next weekend, and I enjoyed it. However, one day during my tea break I was sitting on a low wall, about to tuck into a KitKat (still my favourite snack!) when suddenly a billy goat nudged up behind me and gave me an enormous buck. I flew off the wall and landed face down in a nearby bucket, which was firmly wedged on my head. I couldn't get the thing off – and meanwhile the goat had eaten the whole KitKat, including the silver foil wrapping!

I might have laughed the episode off, but the farmer and my parents agreed that it would be too dangerous for me to continue with the work, because of my medical condition. I had only lasted a month and the job had not made my fortune, since I was paid only seventy pence an hour, but it had been good while it lasted.

Matt soon came up with an alternative plan. He suggested that I sell red worms for bait to the fishing tackle shops, and to members of the local Christchurch Angling Club. I thought it was a slightly revolting idea, but agreed to give it a go.

Matt took me to a wholesale store, where we bought one hundred plastic cups with lids there. At the stables, we dug deep down into the dung heap. We were looking for the moister dung, which was crawling with thousands of tiny red worms. We put them into a big container.

'Anton,' Matt said, 'I would like you to put ten worms in each carton. Then add some light moist horse dung to keep the worms moist'. I went ahead. I began to get quite excited about my new business, and I designed my own adverts, which were fixed to fishing tackle shop windows.

The phone started ringing quite soon after I had distributed my adverts. Many fishing shops called to order worms and I had to get up very early each morning to dig for more in the dung heap at Ashtree. Business boomed from the start. I sold each carton for fifty pence and because my initial outlay was so small I was soon making a lot of profit. However, it was not long before my disability let me down. My hands had swollen up, from gripping the fork handle for so long, and my legs and hips were soon very painful too from all the digging.

I had to give up the work, and my cousin took over. He had an even better idea than selling worms – he decided to sell the dung itself, as garden fertiliser. He did very well, and although I was pleased for him I was frustrated too, because I was so hampered by my disabilities.

As the year went on and I still had no luck finding work, I started to become increasingly stressed, and this manifested in terrible stomach cramps. I had troubles digesting food, and issues with constipation and diarrhoea. I was so miserable.

One day I was so badly constipated, and so dizzy, that I was rushed to hospital, where I was given several enemas – a really embarrassing experience. Mum took matters into her own hands and went to the health food shop to but me a homeopathic remedy. This was called

'Slippery elms', a white powder which could be mixed into a drink to help smooth the digestive tract. I drank it three times a day, and it helped a lot.

I still had cramps though, and so I went to see my GP, who told me I should eat less meat and more fruit and vegetables. This worked – I found that apples especially helped ease the cramps. I felt a lot better, and decided to follow a vegetarian diet, which finally did the trick. Mum soon got the hang of cooking vegetarian food and I felt a lot healthier.

Early in 1982, an old friend, Rog, asked whether I would like to design and construct some signs to advertise Morey's Trucks Agricultural Show, which was held in Ringwood, Hampshire. I jumped at the opportunity, although it was a big challenge.

I started immediately, working every day from 9 am to 4.30pm at my friend's workshop, rubbing down the wooden boards and painting them in white undercoat and gloss. I had just over a hundred small signs to do, for the car park, agricultural machinery, marquees event, toilets, trade stores, show jumping events, as well as four big signs for the Morey's Daf Trucks tower display unit.

I found the work hard going. I was sign writing with a brush, and used plain block lettering, but constant use made my fingers swell and they became very sore. Sometimes I worked alone and listened to to the radio for company. One afternoon I heard that unemployment had reached a record figure in the UK – there were now three million people without jobs!

There were constant news flashes about the situation

with Argentina too – apparently they were threatening to capture the Falkland Islands, which meant that we could soon be at war. I was worried at the prospect, not knowing what it would entail. I hadn't known much about the Falkland Islands up to that point, but listening to the radio as I worked, I found out a lot about the subject.

It was quite complicated, involving all sorts of history and politics, and I did wonder why Britain still exerted sovereignty over the area. As I listened to the radio debate, I discovered that there were a lot of oil, gas and minerals there, which helped to explain matters.

Soon the Argentines landed on South Georgia in the Falklands, which precipitated the war. It was not a popular move – people in the UK were too concerned with their own problems, and the lack of jobs, than in a war over some territory that most people had never heard of before.

But the government, as usual, made our decisions for us, and war it was. Events, once the war started, continued inexorably – with bombers taking off here, destroyers being damaged there... I watched the action unfold on the television throughout the month of April and into May, and I was surprised to find myself feeling quite patriotic, and proud to be British. I was concerned, though, for my sister and her husband – he was in the Royal Navy, and took part in the conflict.

I was sad to be finishing my work for Morey's Daf Trucks agricultural show. I was pleased to have achieved what I set out to do though - I had managed to make all the signs in time. On the last day, just as I was leaving work, I had a surprise visitor – Adam Morey himself, the owner of the business, who thanked me for my work. 'The signs look really professional,' he said. 'You should start your own business, sign writing'.

'Maybe I will one day,' I told him. 'But I wouldn't know where to start just now'.

'Look, Anton,' he said, 'If you ever decide to take the plunge and start your own business, I would be more than happy to help you. Just call me any time'.

I had a free family ticket for the agricultural show, but in the end I decided not to go, because I realised that I would struggle to walk around such a big area.

I was really glad to have had some experience of proper work at last. Now I had something to put on my CV! However, although I re-doubled my efforts to find more paid work, I had no luck.

Meanwhile, May was passing and the Falklands War was still raging. I still watched it on the television, identifying strongly with our troops. I was particularly proud of the Sea Harriers – amazing planes, which I would sometimes see flying over on their way to join the combat.

Incredibly, when the World Cup began on June 13th, England and Argentina enrolled to take part. I was staggered by this in view of what was happening in the Falklands – but the very next day the Argentinians finally flew their white flags and a formal surrender was agreed.

Now I could concentrate on the World Cup, which was always a thrill. Spain was hosting play this year. I still supported Brazil of course, and they had a great new team, with many top players led by their top star Zico. I thought they had an easy group to play against, including the Soviet Union, Scotland and New Zealand. I was still nervous for them, though, and I bit my fingernails to the quick watching those games!

On the 21st June my attention moved closer to home when Prince William, the first child of the Prince and Princess of Wales, was born at St Mary's Hospital in Paddington. Meanwhile, Brazil were playing fantastically, and I had high hopes that they would win the World Cup for the fourth time. It was so exciting! This was not to be, unfortunately – Italy became World Champions. So I set my sights ahead to 1986, hoping that Brazil would win the beautiful game again then, and regain the cup.

On the 21st July I watched the Royal Navy flagship HMS Hermes, docking at Portsmouth to a hero's welcome. Thousands of people were waiting to be reunited with their loved ones. Banners and flags were waved – the messages on the banners varying from the moving 'Welcome Home, Dad' to the hysterical 'Knickers to the Argies!' We all felt very moved, and of course there was a personal aspect to our celebration - Julie's husband was home, safe and sound.

There was a flypast then, from the Harriers, Army Lynx helicopters and Naval Hunter training squadron, accompanying the ageing ship as she cruised into port. The words of Margaret Thatcher came to me as I watched the spectacle, 'I have no regrets'. And for once the mood of the country chimed with that of the Prime Minister.

I identified myself as more British from that point. I may have supported Brazil in the football, but I knew what it was to feel patriotic too – the United Kingdom has an impressive history and wonderful traditions and we are a nation to be proud of.

At that time I bought my first car. It was a Mini Metro. The car was mine on a four year lease, fully paid for with my disability allowance, through the Motability Scheme. This was a marvellous arrangement, as far as I was concerned – the car came fully taxed and insured and the price included a full new set of tyres each year. All I had to do was pay for fuel – and when the lease was up I could get a brand new car. I was thrilled!

A kind neighbour let me keep the car in her garage. I had driving lessons in it, and I practised as much as possible between lessons – friends helped greatly, teaching me the highway code and accompanying me on trips (with my L Plates attached) so I could get more experience. I found learning to drive was very nerve-racking, but at the same time I enjoyed every minute of it.

Mum paid for my driving lessons, as I still had no job – but one day she suggested that I should sign on the dole. I knew she was right, and that I could not expect my Mum and Dad to pay for my keep for ever, so I took her advice, and made my way to the nearby Labour Exchange.

I did not relish the experience at all – I felt quite uncomfortable standing in the long queues. The officials behind their counters looked bored and uninterested when I approached to sign my name. It felt demeaning, as if I was begging for money instead of earning it. It was a disturbing feeling too, to be amongst so many others in the same predicament.

I hated signing on so much, but I kept on going, and as a reward I got £42 each week in dole money. I paid my Mum £35 of this for my keep, which didn't leave me much – but I could take part-time work as long as I didn't earn more than £16 a week, which was some comfort.

In December I took my driving test. I was excited and nervous in equal measure - I was desperate to pass the test, and had got it into my head that I wanted to do so on my first attempt. However, my emergency stop was a disaster. I had noticed that the examiner was not wearing a seat belt before I did the manoeuvre, but when I brought this to his attention he told me to continue regardless. Then during the emergency stop, he bumped his head on the rear view mirror and cut it badly. He had blood dripping all down his face.

It was horrific. But he told me to carry on with the test, so I did. Just then a fire engine screeched up behind us, sirens blaring, and I pulled over to let it pass. 'Why did you stop?' he asked sternly.

'Err, because there was a fire engine which needed to get through,' I told him. I'd thought this was the right thing to do in the circumstances – but after his question, I wasn't sure any more. I made my way back to the test centre, with the examiner still bleeding away, and tried not to look at his wound as we sat outside in the car and he asked me questions about the Highway Code. I had pretty much given up all hope of passing by now.

The   examiner   finally   turned   to   me   smiling.

'Congratulation, Mr Evans,' he said. 'You have passed your driving test. Please wait here in your car for your instructor, who will give you your certificate.'

I literally cried for joy. Mum and Dad were so happy and excited when they heard and I was so pleased and proud – passing my driving test was by far the best Christmas present I'd ever had. Driving a car changed my life in a big way – I still drive today, and I still love every minute of it.

Chapter Twenty
Freedom at Last

The good times began now, with some of the most memorable and enjoyable moments of my life, driving my Motability Mini Metro all over the place. I loved the sense of freedom, and found driving on the busy roads through Christchurch and Bournemouth surprisingly easy. Parking was never a problem, because I had a blue disabled badge fixed to my back windscreen, and this entitled me to park on double yellow lines, and neither did I have to pay in car parks. (These entitlements do not apply to every person with a 'blue badge' – they depend on the severity of the disability.)

I did have to remember to display my disabled ID, and another clock disc card, to notify the traffic warden how long I had parked for. If I went over the three hour limit, I could be booked and have to pay a £30 fine – and I could also be disqualified from Motability, so I was very careful to keep within the rules.

I often went fishing in those days, as a member of Christchurch Angling Club. I found this a relaxing occupation, which helped to take my mind off the stress of being unemployed. My favourite location was a private lake in Ringwood belonging to the club, but one day I had a horrible experience there.

I arrived at the Ringwood lakes early one morning and drove straight to the disabled car park, which was very close to the lakes. I found a nice spot to fish, between the trees, and settled down, finding it very pleasant to listen to the birds singing there.

I set up my fishing gear and started to fish, using

maggots for bait. It was a quiet morning, and I got lucky very quickly – after just an hour I had caught many different sorts of freshwater fish, including roach, chub, carp, and dace.

But suddenly I was approached by two burly fishermen, who demanded to see my fishing licence. I handed it over, and then to my surprise they refused to give it back. Instead they started to shout and swear at me.

'We are not happy with you, short arse,' they said to me. 'You have broken the rules, coming in here too early with your car. Now we are asking you to leave – or else!'

They did not expand on 'what' else, but I knew it wasn't going to be nice. 'I haven't broken any rules,' I said. 'I did not come in too early. Just leave me alone and go and pick on someone your own size, both of you, you big bullies!'

They started to get aggressive then, verbally and physically. I got really upset. Eventually I got totally fed up and threw all my fishing equipment into the lake. 'Are you bloody satisfied now?' I yelled at them.

I was really upset and I stormed off to my car. I drove to the nearest telephone box and rang my Mum. I was shaking and crying by now, with fear and humiliation. My Mum told me to come straight back home, where she made me a cup of tea and told me to rest.

Meanwhile, Mum called a friend of the family, who was a bailiff at the Angling Club, and she told him what had happened to me in Ringwood. Late that afternoon the doorbell rang and our friend was there, holding all my fishing equipment, which was covered in duckweed.

'Hello, Anton,' he said. 'I am so sorry to hear that you were so badly abused this morning. We have expelled the two fishermen from the Club already, and notified the police too. And here is your fishing gear – I dredged it out of the small lake you were fishing in.'

'Why do you think they picked on me?' I asked him.

'I think what happened was that you chose the best fishing spot, and that upset them,' he explained. 'But there really is no excuse for their behaviour. And don't worry, none of this was your fault – you didn't break any rules. I am just so glad that you weren't hurt'.

Later that week I received a letter from the Chairman of the Club, with an official apology. I decided to fish closer to home from then on though, because I didn't want to risk brushing into any other unpleasant fishermen at Ringwood who might try to use me as bait!

I was still applying for jobs, but I still had no luck. I felt a lot of boredom, and I found that the best remedy for this was to drive to the nearby Avon beach, where I sat in my car in the car park, looking out towards the Isle of Wight. I listened to a lot of French music, on RTL, a French radio station, and I was starting to pick up some of the language too, by listening carefully. It was good to keep my mind active.

One day I arrived at the car park very early, about 6am. I sat in my usual spot, watching the sun rise between the headland of the Isle of Wight and the Needles. Early morning is the best time to see the glowing red sun glittering on the sea, backed by the fresh steely blue of the sky.

I switched the car radio to longwave and to my surprise my favourite singer, Demis Roussos, burst out with his hit record, 'Happy to be on an island in the sun'. I felt that this was a marvellous coincidence, since I was sitting watching the sun rise over an island in the distance!

In February of that year I embarked on some voluntary work for the Christchurch and Avon Valley Preservation Society. I was asked to design a logo for the 'Keep Christchurch Green' campaign. I was pleased with my oak tree design, when it was finished. It was used for many display boards around Christchurch and even on T-shirts.

One day, my friend Rog turned up at my house. 'Do you still do photography, Anton?' he asked.

'Well, I'd like to,' I replied. 'But I don't have a camera or an enlarger any more. Why?'.

'Well, I have a building project coming up,' he told me. 'I have to build the new Avonvale Bakery. I need someone to take photos of it as it goes up'.

Rog wanted me to be on site with him every day, taking photographs to show how the new bakery was constructed, from start to finish. He was not going to pay me, but he said he would buy me all the photographic equipment I needed to do the job.

'It's a deal!' I said. 'When do you want me to start?'

'In about two weeks' time,' my friend replied. 'I am just

waiting for a large caravan to arrive on the building site. That will be my office and you can use it too, to take notes if you need to and to do your photography work. Your Dad is going to build you a photographic shed studio in your garden so that you can develop the prints'.

So Rog had already spoken to Dad behind my back and they had sorted out all this between them! I appreciated Rog for doing this though – he knew that I hated being out of work and so he wanted to keep me occupied, to give me a confidence boost.

I started at the Avonvale Bakery site soon afterwards, beginning by taking photos of the builders. One cheeky chap pulled down his trousers and mooned at me. 'Take this for size,' he said. 'You can put it on a builder's calendar for the ladies'.

'If I had my double shot gun,' said Rog, 'I'd shoot him up the a***. That would get him back to work!' I laughed so much, and this set the pattern for the days ahead. Rog had a great sense of humour and often had me in fits with his jokes, often at the expense of the builders.

Each week I spent many hours taking photos and printing them. I really enjoyed it, especially the feeling of being my own boss. When I finished the job, my friend let me keep all the photographic equipment, which was a great bonus.

At that time sciatica, a burning sensation which ran down my leg, which had already been playing up towards the end of the bakery project, became excruciatingly painful. I went downhill fast, and my parents paid for me to have an injection in my spine at a private hospital.

Unfortunately, the procedure did not work. We went through the NHS system the next time, and I went to Southampton Hospital for treatment. They did an investigative procedure, which was a horrific experience – I was strapped face-down to a bed and injected with a red dye, then had to be turned upside down on the bed, so that the dye would travel around my body. My entire body had been numbed with an injection in my spine, so that I could not move while special X-rays were taken.

They did find what was wrong – a trapped nerve – but they said that it would be far too dangerous to operate. If the procedure went wrong, it could result in my death.

I went to see my consultant, Dr Wilkinson, again, to see what else I could do. He said that although he was not officially supposed to recommend a chiropractor, off the record he suggested that I should give it a go.

I was desperate by now. I was living in almost constant agony. So I went to the Anglo European College of Chiropractic in Bournemouth. Again I paid privately, and although I found the procedure embarrassing and uncomfortable (the students who treated me used pressure to relax the sciatic nerve) I was amazed when it worked!

It really was a remarkable result. No drugs had been involved in my treatment – just manipulation of a muscle – and I was pain-free at long last. I was so grateful for this treatment – and although I still occasionally suffer from sciatica today, it can be treated in the same way.

Although physically I felt much better, work-wise I felt

as though I was back at square one. I had nothing to do with my time, and I was finding it hard to cope with the boredom. I was desperate to find a job, or an apprenticeship in graphic design work. One day I decided to take matters into my own hands. There was a big local firm in Christchurch called Mapline Engineering, and although they were not advertising for workers I decided to ask whether they would give me a chance.

I dressed up in my smartest outfit, packed my art portfolio, and drove myself to the engineering firm. When I arrived at Mapline Reception, I waited until a very tall man entered and asked what he could do to help.

I explained to him that I was eager to find work. 'I am well qualified,' I said, 'And I am really keen to work, but I can't seem to get any position, or even find work experience with a graphic design company. I get turned down all the time'.

'You have come to the right place,' he told me. 'We don't have any graphic design vacancies, but we could retrain you to do other design work'.

'I'll take anything,' I said quickly.

'I'll show you around the place and explain,' he said. 'Then we can have a chat with my colleague'.

Grant, who turned out to be the manager of the firm, showed me around. There was a huge room filled with student designers, working on their drawing boards, designing printed circuit boards, and illustrating buildings in technical graphics. Next Grant took me into his office to meet Joe, his colleague, and talk about a training course. 'We do cater for disabled people here, Anton,' Grant reassured me. 'It's part of our job to make sure that the working conditions are suitable for you. I would like to offer you the opportunity to become a designer – you choose your preferred field'.

I could hardly believe my luck. 'I think,' Grant went on, 'That because you are skilled at drawing and art in general, we could retrain you to do architectural design and planning. We could also teach you how to do dye line printing to print your plans. And we could give you a grounding in knowledge of basic building materials – house bricks, concrete blocks, residential roofing, concrete roofing and tiles'.

'It all sounds great,' I said. 'But how will it work? How long will the course last? And what about money? Will I still need to sign on?'

'You won't be signing on the dole any more,' Grant told me. 'This is a government scheme, and they will pay you to train – almost the same amount as you get from signing on. They pay us too, to train you'.

Grant explained all the details, and when he finished speaking I nodded and smiled, and we shook hands on the deal. I rushed home – I was so excited to tell my Mum and Dad all about it! Mum was wary at first, 'What sort of work did they offer you, Antony?' she asked.

I showed Mum and Dad the printed information that Grant had given me, and they agreed that it looked like a promising opportunity. 'Are you happy to do another course though?' asked Mum. 'Are you guaranteed to get a job afterwards?'

'It's got to be better than signing on the dole,' I told her. 'At the very least I'll get work experience'.

Mum was still cautious, but after ringing Mapline Engineering and speaking to Grant, she was reassured. She and Dad agreed that I should go ahead, and said that they were both really proud of me for setting myself up with this training course.

I was delighted the next day when I went to the Purewell Labour Exchange to sign off the dole. It was such a relief to know that I would not have to go there weekly any more!

My first day at Mapline Engineering soon dawned. When I arrived I was given a space in the huge room that Grant had shown me around on my previous visit. I was set up with a large drawing board fixed to a stand, with a swivel desk chair and a studio storage desk near to the window, with the other retrained designers.

I had dressed smartly for work in black trousers, white shirt and a green tie. My first assignment, for the first month of training, was to create and design a printed circuit board. This was quite a learning curve – there was a whole new language to learn, quite aside from the technical ability. Grant was helpful throughout, coming to my rescue whenever I ran into problems.

The second part of my course was even more challenging, as there was a lot of Maths involved. I learned architectural design and had to study many different types of building materials. Drawing roof tiles was especially difficult and next I progressed to drawing window frames, doors and many other parts of buildings, none of which came to me any more easily. I was glad when this part of the course came to an end too – I had learned a great deal, but I had realised that it was not the career path for me.

I met with Grant, who said that I was doing well and that he and Joe were glad that I was persevering with the course. 'I have some good news for you,' Grant told me then. 'I have had a letter from your sister, asking whether you can take a day off work. She has arranged for you to visit the Royal Navy Fleet Yeovilton Air Station. I believe you are going to see the Sea Harrier Jump Jet'.

I was really excited to hear this! 'Julie knows that the Harrier is my favourite aircraft!' I told Grant. 'It was used in the Falklands war, you know. It was designed to hover'.

'I know,' said Grant. 'I like them too. In fact I'm jealous – I wish I could go with you! How did your sister manage to fix it?'

'She works in Defence,' I said.

'A handy woman to know then,' he said. 'You really are lucky'.

Early the next day I met Julie at the main entrance of the Royal Navy Fleet Air Station. She introduced me to a naval officer who gave me a special pass with my name on. It was extremely exciting – one of my favourite dreams was about to come true. I was about to see my favourite aircraft up close!

The airfield runway was very busy and extremely noisy, with Sea King helicopters hovering above us as we entered the hangar. I was scared, but I forgot all that when I saw the aircraft in front of me. There it was at last – the Sea Harrier Jump Jet FRS1.

The Harrier looked massive. It was less than perfect though – it was one of the aircraft which had returned from the Falklands, had been hit by several bullets on its tail end, and was having major repairs. I asked the officer why the aircraft was painted grey, and he told me that it was for camouflage. He said that in the Falklands the weather was often overcast with grey sky, so the grey of the aircraft blended in with the grey skies.

I was shown around inside the Harrier then, and introduced to two more naval officers who were waiting near the cockpit. Then I had the biggest surprise ever, when one of the officers asked whether I would like to sit in the cockpit!

Would I ever?! I don't think I could have been more excited if I had tried, but I managed to contain myself as I was helped to climb up a small ladder, from which I lowered myself into the cockpit. This was an amazing experience – I knew that there were few people in the world who had had the pleasure of such an experience!

I was given an aircraft helmet to wear, with a special visor attached, marked with grid lines. It looked very high tech, and suddenly I felt convinced that I could take off in this wonderful Sea Harrier and fly back to land it in my back garden. If only! I imagined myself in Thunderbird Two, ready for take off. 'FAB' I said to myself. 'Thunderbirds are Go!'

Unfortunately it was soon time for me to leave, but I had one last great experience. As I exited the hangar, there was a parade of Sea Harriers hovering in the sky, doing their training exercises. It was a wonderful thing to watch, as they hovered and slowly landed and took off again, climbing vertically up into the sky.

Finally the planes roared off into the sky, disappearing into the low grey clouds until all that was left was the mighty rumble of their engines. It was a brilliant performance, and a fantastic ending to my day.

I hugged my sister goodbye, and thanked her for organising the special day out. As I drove back home I imagined myself back in the Sea Harrier cockpit, but unfortunately I eventually had to accept that I was driving my Mini Metro car, on four ordinary wheels. When I got back I was feeling really tired and poorly, and as it happened I went down with flu the next day and couldn't return to Mapline Engineering for many weeks afterwards.

I was so ill. I ached all over, and was so weak that I couldn't get out of bed. The GP paid me many home visits, but all he could do was to tell me to drink plenty of water. He thought I might have contracted the virus at the Navy Fleet Air Station.

It took five weeks before I was ready to return to work, and when I got back I found that lots of others had come down with the flu too, and were still off work. Joe was pleased to see me back, and he called me into his office for a chat.

'How are you feeling, Anton?' he asked.

'Much better, thanks,' I said.

'Grant and I want to ask for your help,' he said then. 'We have a sixteen year old from Bournemouth School for Boys, who is with us on a work placement. Because we are short of staff due to the flu virus, we are wondering whether you would step in. We want you to teach him how to draw his parents' bungalow'.

I started on this new project the following week, taking photos of the boy's house, which I used to help him make a technical drawing. We finished the illustrations the following week.

Joe called me into his office and reassured me that helping Alex would count as part of my training. He said that I had done it brilliantly. 'I am really pleased,' he told me, 'And I am sure that Grant will be too'.

It was almost May now, and I only had two months of the training course left. The days ticked by faster than I could keep track of them. One day Joe asked me to drive to Burley, in the New Forest, to take some photographs of Burley Manor. Later I printed the photos and showed them to Grant so that he could decide which ones I should use for my drawing. While we were looking at the photos together, Grant told me that he'd had a letter from the headteacher of Bournemouth School for Boys, saying that they were very impressed with my drawing skills and with how I had helped Alex with his bungalow design. 'Well done again, Anton,' Grant told me, and I was very proud.

Grant instructed me to draw Burley Manor in a technical illustration 3D effect. I was learning fast, and enjoyed using this new kind of technique. The 3D illustration took me nearly three weeks to finish, and Joe and Grant said that I had created an excellent building design.

There was just one month left of my course at Mapline. One morning I was asked to find an 'important house' to draw in technical graphics. Grant said that he would like me to use my own technique skills, as before, and that I had four weeks to complete the work. He required me to do two drawings, of the front and rear elevations.

I enjoyed a challenge, and this was certainly a challenge! But how would I find an 'important building' to draw, I wondered? I started to panic a little, thinking hard about what I could do.

I drove my car out to the New Forest, heading towards Donkey's Bottom. Somewhere at the back of my mind I could remember picnicking there with my family as a teenager, and I vaguely remembered a big house nearby.

When I arrived I soon saw the house I remembered, and started to drive very slowly along the long driveway that led to it. It was a beautiful house, with many trees and large grass lawns surrounding it. I made my way to the main door and nervously rang the bell.

A very posh looking chap opened the door, and asked politely how he could help me. I introduced myself, and asked nervously whether I could draw his house, and to my pleasure he agreed. He told me that his name was Mr Meyrick. He called his gardener, and I explained that I would like to take photos of the house. The gardener asked whether he could have a copy of my drawing when it was completed. 'I can use it as a guide line for new flower beds,' he said.

273

'Of course,' I replied.

I walked around the gardens, taking many wide angle shots of the front and back of the house, and after a while two women approached me, dressed in tennis gear. 'Hello,' said one of them. 'I'm Mr Meyrick's daughter, and this is my friend. Is there any chance you could take a photo of us by the tennis court?'

I took the photos as they wanted, and then they invited me to sit in the garden and have a cream tea with them. 'What a lovely name you have,' said one. 'Where did you get it? Is it French?'

'It is,' I replied. 'A friend gave it to me'.

'Very sweet,' she said. 'Do you live locally, Anton?'

'In Purewell,' I replied. 'I sometimes stay at my Grandads' house, Ashtree Riding School'.

'Gosh,' said the lady, 'I go riding there myself. What a lovely place your family have!'

I finished the photos and headed off home, thinking what a splendid day it had been, meeting Mr Meyrick and Tom and the two pretty ladies. Back at Mapline the remainder of the week was very busy, as I copied my photos into illustrations of the house. I completed my drawing of Mr Meyrick's house well within the allocated time and I drove out to the house and gave Tom two copies of the drawings, which he thanked me for.

It was soon my last day at Mapline, and time to say goodbye and thank you to Grant and Joe. They handed me a certificate which confirmed that I had completed the six month course. I should have been happy, but by the time I got home that evening I was instead feeling very low. I talked to my Mum about it, saying that I felt I was back at the beginning again – no job and no occupation. 'Don't worry son,' she said. 'You just have to keep trying. It will all turn out okay in the end'.

Chapter Twenty-One
Purewell Signwriters

It was the end of the summer now. My confidence had fallen since I had found myself out of work again, but I refused to sign on the dole, although I could have done with the money. I did manage to make a few pennies – I created books and posters, photos and cards, but I didn't much like selling them, and so profits were minimal.

In September Mum spoke to a very kind lady, who helped disabled people to set up their own small businesses. I showed her my two art portfolios, full of photographic work and illustrations, and she said that in her opinion I was very talented indeed. 'Why don't you set up your own business?' she asked.

'I wouldn't know where to start,' I replied.

'Ah, well I can help you with that,' she told me.

And she did help. She set me up on a two week business training course in Bournemouth. All the others stayed at the hotel for the duration of the course, but I travelled in daily. We all bonded, had good fun and learned a lot about VAT, accounting and customer service. Everybody had a business plan – I remember that one lady wanted to set up a land train along the Bournemouth Sea Front – but I am not sure how many of these ideas saw fruition.

My birthday took place during the course, but I don't remember much about it. The rest of that year is a bit of a blur in my memory too. We had Grandad's tea party on Christmas Day as usual, but nothing else really stands out in my mind.

I remember those last months of 1984 in a positive light though. At last I had a focus, a mission – I had decided that I would start my own business, and I was really excited about it. I had a lot of research to do, but I had a feeling that somehow things were going to turn out just fine.

I had learned a lot from the small business course. All I had to work out now was exactly what sort of business I wanted to create. Meanwhile I went to Pimpernel Press and asked them if they could make me a large rubber stamp, with my name and 'Freelance Graphic Designer' on it. The idea was that I could use this to stamp in black ink onto my letter heads – it had the potential to save me a fortune in stationery!

A friend soon asked me to do some freelance work, so I found a signwriter in Bournemouth. His name was Paddy, and he was a very congenial type of person. We soon established that we could work together. 'I need a double sided pavement sign made, for a hair salon,' I said. 'Can you give me a quote?' He named a price, which I then added an extra amount to, so that I could make a small profit. I saw my friend the next day, and he readily agreed to the price.

I went to the nearest public phone box to call Paddy, to tell him to go ahead. However I hit a big problem here – the handset was too high for me to reach! I asked a passing lady to help, and she was very kind, dialling the number for me, and telling me to take as long as I needed on the call and that she would then replace the handset.

I spoke to Paddy, who thanked me for the order and said

that he would have the board ready by the end of the week. Then I gave the handset back to the lady and thanked her for her help. 'No need to thank me,' she said. 'I just wish that British Telecom would make their phone boxes easier for you to use'.

When I got home I told my Mum and Dad what had happened at the phone box. Mum said that she had read in the paper that day that BT were going to phase out the old red boxes, and replace them with smaller versions. And they soon did − but to my disgust lots of small villages were loathe to see them go, and bought the boxes privately so that they could continue using them. I hated the things − reminders of my humiliation that they were!

A week later I got the call from Paddy to say that the hairdresser's 'A board' was finished and ready for collection. I drove to his studio in Bournemouth, and found a narrow parking space outside. I managed to squeeze in between two other cars, and found that when I got out of my vehicle a traffic warden was standing staring at me. 'Sorry Sir,' I said. 'Did you want me to move?'

'Not at all,' he said. 'I am just amazed at how you managed to reverse into that tiny parking space'.

'Well, I have a good brain,' I replied jokingly, and he laughed and said that I certainly must have.

I delivered the board to my friend, who was very pleased with it. That night I found it hard to get to sleep, although I could not put my finger on why. Something was bugging me. I just lay on my back on the bed, staring at the ceiling, and my mind wouldn't switch off and let me rest. I felt as though someone was trying to tell me something.

The next morning I drove to Bournemouth town centre, parked up, and watched all the people walking in and out of the various shops.

The time drifted on. I sat there for hours, quite enjoying the spectacle. Then suddenly it came to me. 'That's it!' I thought. 'People need signs and logos for their shop windows and displays!' I realised then what I was going to do – I was going to start a business in signwriting!

I went to see Paddy again, and asked whether he would be willing to work as my subcontractor, and he agreed immediately. I then decided that I needed to find another signwriter, who could do commercial vehicles, boats and so on. I put an advert in the paper and had many replies from people desperate for the job. It was nice to be on the other side for a change!

I interviewed many people, but was disappointed to find that most of them could not spell, or even read properly, and that their portfolios were disappointing. One afternoon though, I had a visit from a young man called Tod. His work was top class, so I gave him the job.

Now I just had two more things to sort out – a place and a name for my business. I decided on the name first, based on the area where I lived. I called it 'Purewell Signwriters' and adopted the logo of a well, after checking that no other local traders used this name or logo.

I now had to find a studio where I could make my signs and carry out my graphic design work. Grandad came to my rescue here – he offered the top of his big barn to me. The ground floor was already in use, by the liveries, who kept their horses there and used it to store tack and feed.

First the barn would need a new staircase, and plenty of other renovation work. Grandad was very generous – he offered to pay half of the cost for the loft conversion and to have an electric meter installed. He also said that he would not charge me rent. I could see my new future shining brightly ahead of me – although I knew that I would have to put in a good deal of work.

I was worried about the cost of setting up the business. I had heard about the Enterprise Allowance scheme set up by the Government, and so I rang up to make an appointment at the local government office to talk about this. I qualified for the allowance, which was great news. 'But what would happen if my business failed after a year?' I asked. 'Would I have to pay all the money back?'

'No,' I was told. 'If things don't work out for you, that will be a shame, but you would not have to pay back any of the Enterprise Allowance money'.

Later that evening my old friend Rog appeared at my front door. 'What are you doing here?' I asked, and Mum laughed. 'Dad and I asked Rog to come over to discuss the loft conversion at Grandad's barn,' she said.

Dad and Rog organised the details of the work together. The next day Rog started building the new staircase to the barn loft. Later on that week his workers arrived at the barn to insulate the walls and put new flooring down. Then an electrician came to install the new electric meter, the studio lights, light switches and power sockets. Finally I had to get the loft decorated. My cousin volunteered to paint the walls white to let more light into the room. It looked great.

At last everything was in place, and to celebrate I invited many local shop traders and other small companies to join the official opening of Purewell Signwriters. Mum supplied all the refreshments, and many people turned up from all over Bournemouth and Christchurch to wish me luck. I was very excited, and also a little nervous at the prospect of getting squashed by all the crowds!

I then made a quick speech. 'I am so happy,' I began, 'That I can finally see the beginning of my dream to be a professional artist! I would like to thank all of you for your help and encouragement, especially my parents and grandparents. I would also like to thank all the tradesmen, and especially Rog, for working so hard on renovating my new barn studio. I would like to announce that Purewell Signwriters is now officially open!'

After the party finished, the proprietor of Pimpernel Press delivered my new business stationery. Rog was still there, and my Dad asked him how much overtime we owed him for the extra work he had done, and the extra supplies he had given us.

'You don't have to give me a thing, Jim,' he replied. 'It is my way of saying thank you to Anton for the marvellous job he did for me on the Avonvale Bakery photographs. I am so proud that he has finally become a professional artist'.

Dad and I were speechless with gratitude. Then I said, 'I bet you won't say no to this Rog'. I held out some gifts we had bought for him – five boxes of his favourite cigars and a large bottle of his favourite tipple, Glenfiddich Scotch Whisky.

Rog gave a big grin. 'Now you're talking, Evans,' he said.

One lunchtime, Dad arrived home from work and said that he had some news for me. 'I have been working at the Royal Exeter Hotel,' he announced, 'And the manager there would like some signs made. Could you call him?'

I rang the Exeter Hotel straight away, and arranged to see the manager, Mr Jones, the following week. I also rang Mr Adam Morey from Daf's Trucks, because I remembered that he had promised to give me some designing work if I ever set up my own designing business. Mr Morey sounded really pleased to hear from me again. 'Have you got any transport?' he asked.

'Yes,' I said. 'I passed my driving test, and I have my own car now'.

'I need a logo for my letterheads and business cards,' he said. 'Can you pop over and see me next week to talk it over?'

'Of course I can,' I said. 'It's no problem at all'. I was really pleased that my new business was getting off to a flying start!

One evening, Uncle Matt was invited to his friend Margaret's birthday party, which was to be held at a hotel in Bournemouth. He invited me to go along with him. The hotel ballroom was very crowded, beautifully decorated, and all the disco equipment was set up on the stage, ready to go.

However, behind the scenes the owners of the hotel were panicking. They had just heard that the DJ they had booked had been taken ill, and it was too late to find someone else to do the music and entertainment. Margaret came over to our table. 'You've got a good sense of humour, Matt,' she said. 'Could you be our DJ for the evening? As a favour to me?'

'Afraid it's not my thing,' Matt replied. 'But I know just the man for you'. He looked at me, smiling encouragingly.

'Uh-uh,' I said. 'No way!'

'But you love music, Anton,' he said. 'And you know so much about it'.

'Please, Anton,' begged Margaret. 'Otherwise this party will turn into a nightmare. I'll pay you well'.

'I'll give it a go,' I said finally. 'But don't blame me if the whole thing goes pear-shaped'.

Luckily I knew how to operate the disco equipment, because of our Jubilee Street party some years before, when I had been the DJ. I had just two minutes to prepare myself and work out how to speak through the microphone and how to operate the controls and turntables. I stayed calm, and managed to find an index book, showing me the names of all the artists whose music they had, in case anyone requested a record.

I was very nervous, a bit shaky about the thought of taking centre stage in front of so many people. The owner came up to me, with a young girl in tow. 'This is Lisa,' he said. 'She is one of my waitresses, and will help you with your music. Thanks so much for stepping into the breach. Good luck!'

Lisa told me not to worry too much, and that she had done disco work before. 'Have you DJ'd before?' she asked.

'No,' I answered, 'This is my first time. I hope all my words come out in the right order, and that I don't make an idiot of myself'.

'You'll be fine,' she reassured me, but I was having a flashback to the time when I had been on stage at Twynham School, ready to play the piano, but had suddenly dried up in front of everybody.

Suddenly, the lights on the dance floor were dimmed. 'This is it, Anton,' whispered Lisa. 'Good luck!'

I decided that I might as well just enjoy it, and I raised the microphone and spoke clearly into it. 'Good evening, everyone,' I said. 'Welcome to Margaret's 50th birthday party. I'm Anton Evans, your replacement disc jockey. Sorry about the last one, who has been suddenly taken ill. Apparently, he's slipped a disc'.

Everybody burst out laughing and I relaxed a little. Then I began the music and encouraged people to get up and dance. I got lots of requests, and the highlight was when one lady asked whether I had a record of Demis Roussos 'Forever and Ever' - I felt that this was a really positive sign that the evening was going to turn out well!

When the party was over I was completely shattered. Everyone gave me a loud cheer, and the owner of the hotel handed me a bottle of Martini Asti, my favourite tipple. Margaret offered me some money for DJ-ing, but I refused to accept it, insisting that I'd really enjoyed the experience.

A few days later, it was April 5th at last - time to start my first day at work in my own business! My first customer was Mr Jones, manager of the Royal Exeter Hotel. Mr Jones showed me around the hotel, to give me an idea of the sort of signs he would need. It was a huge project. And the hotel was not just having new signs – it was having an entire makeover, so I would not be the only tradesman called in to work.

I spent many hours with Mr Jones, discussing the best signs to have in the public areas. He asked for a quote to be delivered as soon as possible, so that he could forward it to the hotel owners. I rushed home, and immediately contacted my two signwriters and Purewell Timbers to get prices for the wood, paints, and so on. That evening I did many calculations, wanting to come up with a reasonable price on which I could earn some profit.

The next morning I drove to the hotel at 7am and handed my quote over. Mr Jones then said that he also needed Christmas signs. 'I need a very large cut-out of Father Christmas too,' he said, 'Riding in his sleigh. That one's going to go on the roof. It needs to be sixteen feet long and four feet high. All in colour with good detail please, and I'll need the quotes as soon as possible again'.

'I'm pretty sure,' he continued, 'Looking at your quote for the first job, that you've got it, and that you'll get the next one too. You don't need to start work until the end of the year, though, because the hotel is going to be closed for three months, for all the other work to be carried out. It's having a complete overhaul'.

I headed towards home light-headed with excitement. But on impulse I stopped at the Lansdowne, at the Roundhouse Hotel where Ellie and I had spent such happy times. I was sitting on the wall of the hotel, thinking of Ellie and our first meeting, when a lady suddenly came up to me and called me by name. I looked at her in confusion.

'Don't you know me, Anton?' she asked. 'I'm Charlie, Ellie's friend'. I was amazed – it had to be fate that I should meet her there at just that moment.

We sat together on the wall, looking towards Royal London House, where we had been at college all those years ago. 'What are you doing now, Charlie?' I asked.

'I am a fashion designer,' she told me. 'I work in Windsor. I'm just down to visit my parents. What are you up to? You look very smart'.

'Well,' I said, 'I have just started my own business in signs and graphics'. I found it hard to keep the pride out of my voice. 'I've just had a meeting with the manager of the Royal Exeter Hotel, about some work. And funnily enough I just stopped here on impulse, to have a think about Ellie'.

'Do you still miss Ellie?' her friend asked me.

'I do,' I confessed. 'I still love her. But it is time for me to move on now. I don't know whether I will ever see her again'.

Charlie told me that if she ever heard from her, she would tell me straight away. 'That's a promise, Anton,' she said. We parted then, and my heart felt a little lighter, because I had spoken to someone about how I felt, and she had understood.

I had designed the stationery for Adam Morey by now, and when I showed my Mum the cheque she was very impressed. 'You'll soon be a millionaire, Anton, if you get a few of those coming in each week' she told me.

It was my 27th birthday that year, and Mum made me a special cake, which tasted as good as it looked. In November I started on the Christmas signs for the Royal Exeter, and they all turned out very well, especially Father Christmas with his reindeer. Uncle Matt delivered everything to the hotel for me, and he reported back that Mr Jones had been so impressed that he was dumbstruck!

That year Grandad had decided to have a New Year's Party, instead of his traditional Christmas one. He said that everyone needed cheering up – the recession was drawing to a close at last, thank goodness, but Grandad felt that everyone was worn out and needed a treat. He announced that I would be DJ-ing for the party, and he also ordered me to go out and buy two enormous Christmas trees, 'The biggest you can find' he said. 'Take your cousin Rich with you to collect them'.

I called Rich. 'What on earth does he want two

enormous trees for?' he grumbled. 'Has he been on the whisky?' The next day, Rich and I went to a garden centre to buy the trees. They were each over ten feet tall, and we struggled to get them to Ashtree House, tying them to the roof rack of my car with heavy rope. It looked as though we were in an army camouflage vehicle, and it wasn't easy to see where we were going. Everybody we passed on the way fell into fits of laughter.

When we finally reached Ashtree House, we had to drag the trees through the house, putting one in the lounge and the other in the sun lounge. Uncle Matt helped, standing the trees up in two plastic dustbins. Grandad came in to look.

'Ha!' he said. 'Call those trees? They're miniscule!'

'You cheeky old thing!' exclaimed Rich, not realising that Grandad was winding us up as usual.

The party took place as scheduled, and it was a full house – all Grandad's friends and family were there, and his staff and all their families too. I hired out a PA system from Jarvis Radio, and took care of the music, acting as DJ. This had been a great year, I thought to myself as I announced to everyone at the stroke of midnight, 'Happy New Year, one and all'. Roll on 1986!

1986 did roll on, and I went to see Mr Jones at the Royal Exeter Hotel about the signs I had promised to make. Mr Jones, the manager, told me that the owners had now decided to replace every sign in the hotel. 'It's a lot more work,' he said. 'Including cartoon menu signs for our new burger kiosk. You'll have to come up with a new quote'.

Just then my Mum phoned. 'Anton, I've just had a call from that hotel in Bournemouth where you did the disco,' she said. 'They want to know whether you can DJ there tonight, between 7pm and midnight'.

I told her that I would do it, and asked her to call the hotel to tell them. Things were getting busy! Mr Jones told me that I could come back the next morning, and since it was already 6pm I found a takeaway nearby, bought myself some dinner, and sat in my car to eat it.

The manager of the hotel was waiting to greet me. 'Thanks so much for coming to our aid again, Anton,' he said. 'You brought the house down with your last disco. They haven't stopped talking about you since. Good luck for tonight by the way – not that you'll need it!'

I felt a tap on my shoulder then, and I spun around. It was Lisa, the waitress, ready to help me with the disco again. The occasion that evening, she told me, was a stag party.

We got stuck into the disco. Soon a beautiful blonde lady wearing a big fur coat walked up to me. 'Hi, DJ babe,' she said. 'I'm going to perform now. Can you put my music on and dim the lights down, please?'

Lisa looked over at me, and laughed at the dumbfounded expression on my face. 'She's a stripper,' she told me. 'She's going to dance for Andrew, the groom'. Poor Andrew looked totally embarrassed as his mates dragged him over to the front of the stage. I put the strip tease tape on, and the girl started to take off her coat in time with the music.

At the crucial moment, Lisa turned the lights off completely. The room was pitch black for about twenty seconds. When Lisa turned the lights back on the stripper was nowhere to be seen. This was clearly part of the act, and Andrew looked very relieved.

At the end of the evening, the manager paid me eighty pounds, of which I gave half to Lisa. It was already half an hour after midnight, and I was tired. Lisa asked if I could give her a lift home – she lived in Southbourne, which was on the way back to my house, so I agreed readily. I soon drew up outside Lisa's house, and turned to say goodnight to her. She was quiet for a minute and then she burst out, 'Anton, would you take me out sometime? You know, on a date?'

It was a very flattering offer. 'I would love to, Lisa,' I told her, 'But I can't.' And then I explained to her about Ellie, who I still loved, although I didn't know whether I would ever see her again. Lisa was very upset, and started to apologise. I reassured her that there was no need to be sorry, and that I thought she was a very lovely person. We agreed to be good friends then, and parted on a high note.

I was exhausted by the time I got home. Mum had left a note on the kitchen table to say that Mr Jones had the plans, and that he needed to see me at the hotel first thing in the morning. I fell into bed then – my hips and legs were very painful from the long and hard day's work I had done.

At eight thirty the next morning I could hardly keep my eyes open at the breakfast table. 'Are you okay, Anton?' Mum asked. 'Your clothes smelt awful – I had to put them all in the washing machine this morning. It must have been very smoky at that disco last night. How did it go, by the way?'

'It was fine,' I said, 'Apart from the smoke. There was a stripper.'

'I bet you enjoyed that,' said Dad.

'She went like a flash,' I told him, and Mum looked puzzled.

'What do you mean?' she asked.

'You don't want to know,' I told her. I finished my eggs and bacon then, and went out to work.

I got to the hotel and was shown straight in to see Mr Jones, who went through all the plans for the new signs with me. There were more than 450 signs to make! 'What do you think?' he asked. I made some quick calls to Purewell Paints and Purewell Timbers and to Paddy and Todd, then I worked out a new quotation on the spot and showed it to Mr Jones. It seemed like an awful lot of money to me, but he readily agreed to pay it. I told Mr Jones that I would need a big deposit for the materials, with the balance to be paid on completion of the work. 'That's fine,' he replied. 'You'd better get cracking then!'

Around that time, my Grandad's housekeeper asked whether I had any painting and decorating work – her son Andy was well qualified but was struggling to find work. He came to see me, and I asked him if he would take on the job of painting the hotel sign boards. 'I need a good professional finish, mind,' I told him.

Andy said that he would be delighted to take on the work. We started together soon afterwards. I was working to a deadline – the signs all had to be ready and delivered by the Easter holidays. I soon started to panic, because February was a very cold month, and although we were on schedule, the paint was taking too long to dry so the signwriting (Paddy and Todd's part of the work) was delayed.

I phoned Mr Jones, to keep him informed of the difficulties I was facing. 'Don't worry,' he said, 'We're not opening for Easter now. We've postponed the opening until the end of May, in fact. The electricians and decorators are behind schedule too.'

'Thank goodness for that!' I said.

'Good luck, Anton,' he said. 'I'll see you again soon'.

I put the phone down with a huge sense of relief, and relayed the good news to my workers. I would have felt awful letting Mr Jones down – he was such a good and decent man.

One evening Grandad sent for me. When I arrived at Ashtree House, he said without preamble, 'How would you like to run your own disco, Anton?'

'Are you serious?' I asked. 'The equipment will cost a fortune. And how will I carry it and rig it up by myself?'

'I'll pay for the equipment,' said Grandad, 'And your cousin Rich says he'll help you'.

I accepted gratefully, and Rich and I soon got lots of disco work. I found it hard to fit it all in at times –

especially keeping up with the Top 40 charts, which meant that I constantly had to buy new records to replenish my stock.

In May I delivered the hotel signs as I had promised, and Mr Jones was very pleased. He said that I could have a party at the Royal Exeter any time, free of charge, so I filed that information away for future reference.

In July I did a big disco for the Mudeford Sandbanks Beach Hut Association. The 'Allo 'Allo themed party was on Mudeford Spit, opposite Mudeford Harbour. We used generators for electricity, because there is no mains electricity there, although families can sleep in the huts. We had a fantastic time - there was music and dancing late into the evening. The only downside was that we had to wait until 3am until we could journey home, because the last ferry had left and we were cut off from the Hengistbury Head road home by the tide.

The next morning, Mum had arranged a surprise outing for me – to Osborne House on the Isle of Wight to see the art collection there. Usually I would really have appreciated this gesture, but this morning I was exhausted and literally had to drag myself out of bed to get ready for the day out!

When we arrived at Osborne House we joined a group of others for a guided tour of the building. The tour guide was showing us what he said was an original Renaissance painting, on loan from the Queen's Collection, but when I looked at it closely, I saw something odd around the border of the picture.

'That's not an original painting at all!' I called out loudly. 'It's a print!'

Mum was seriously embarrassed, and so was the tour guide, who carried on with his talk, trying to ignore me. When he had finished his talk, he called me over and asked me to accompany him to the office. I did so, wondering what I had let myself in for. But all he said was that I was right, and the painting was indeed a print, and that I had done well to spot it. There was no explanation for why he had talked the painting up in the first place.

Several weeks later a letter arrived from Osborne House, addressed to me. In the letter was a job offer – I was asked if I would like to be a tour guide myself! I turned the position down, although I was flattered to have been offered it and I would have liked to work with art. I knew it would be impractical – too far to travel, and anyhow I already had plenty of work.

It seemed ironic really, that I had spent so long trying to find work, and now I had my own signwriting business, my own disco business and I was being solicited for other work too!

Chapter Twenty-Two
Gnomes, the Great Storm, and Grandad

By August I was worn out and had to rest for a month, on doctor's orders. I had strained my body by overworking, and had serious leg pains and dizzy spells. The doctor said that this was nature's warning and that I should take it seriously.

In September I had my first experience of flying, in my Great-Uncle's aeroplane. We flew from Hurn Airport near Christchurch over to the Isle of Wight. We then landed again near his home in New Milton, Hampshire. I hated the whole thing – it was a terrifying, horrible experience, and I never wanted to do it again!

I was 28 in October, and celebrated by watching Neighbours, my favourite Australian soap. I still watch that programme every day after my lunch!

This year, Grandad had planned a big New Year's Party. Rich and I did the disco, and at Grandad's request we had to end, as always, with the National Anthem. The party was a huge success, packed with Grandad's family and friends. He was getting frail by now, and I think we all suspected that it might be the last big party he threw. At the end of the evening, after the National Anthem, I led everyone in a toast to Grandad, to thank him for the party and wish him a Happy New Year. We had certainly seen it in with a bang!

1987 started well for me - my business was flourishing. One morning, I had a call from a pensioner who asked whether I could refurbish her four garden gnomes. I thought this would be a quick and easy job, but I got a shock when I went to collect the gnomes – they were over three feet tall each, and very heavy indeed!

I worked in Mrs White's conservatory, first using a wire brush to take off the green mould which coated all the gnomes, then giving them a base coat of white acrylic paint. I then spent the rest of the week restoring them to their original glory, with pink faces, black trousers, red top hoods, blue waistcoats and white shirts. To cap it off I coated the gnomes with clear varnish, which gave them a sparkle and made them waterproof.

'Oh Anton!' Mrs White declared when she saw the finished job, 'You've brought them back to life again! What a clever chap you are. I've made us a cream tea to celebrate – it's ready for us in the lounge'.

I followed her out to the lounge, and was taken aback to find the room full of people – she'd invited all her friends to see the refurbished gnomes and to meet me. One old lady was pouring the tea. 'Are you a TIF or a MIF?' she asked me, and I replied without missing a beat, 'MIF and one lump of sugar please'.

The lady looked at me, impressed. 'You are one of us,' she said approvingly.

I had only known what she had meant because I'd happened to watch a programme about the Queen on TV. They'd shown her speaking to her butler, who'd asked, 'TIF or MIF, Ma'am?' and the voice over had explained that this was code for 'Tea In First or Milk In First?'

I'd stored away the knowledge, never thinking that it would come in useful for impressing a meeting of the Gnome Appreciation Society! I had a lovely cream tea, and got lots of orders from the other pensioners, to refurbish their gnomes. I felt a bit overwhelmed by this – but decided that it was better to keep them happy than to leave them 'Moaning' – or should I say, 'Gnoming'?

Early one spring morning I came downstairs for breakfast to find that Mum had been crying. 'What's wrong?' I asked. Dad said Grandad had been taken ill the night before, and was now in the hospital. 'We don't know what's wrong yet,' he said. 'We're just waiting for test results'.

I was very upset. I went out to my barn studio to work on my signs, hoping it would take my mind off matters. I found it hard to concentrate though – I sat looking over at Ashtree House through the barn window, hoping against hope that Grandad would be alright.

Eventually my cousin Rich arrived, and said that I should go with him to Ashtree House. When we arrived we found the whole family assembled there. Mum gave a little speech, 'Thank you all for coming over at such short notice,' she started. 'I am very sorry and sad to announce that my father has lung cancer, and the hospital have told us that he only has a short time to live'.

Mum said that we should all carry on as normal, since this was what my Grandad wanted. He was allowed to come home, she said, but would be looked after by the family twenty-four hours a day, with a back-up nurse.

We were all in shock. We felt devastated – Grandad and Ashtree House were the flagship of the family, and we knew instinctively that when he was gone things would change beyond recognition. I gave Mum a hug, and told her that I was going over to my studio because I needed to be on my own. When I got there I looked out of the window as usual towards Ashtree House, and I began to cry. I felt very lost and alone, but I knew that I would have to do my best to be strong, for my mother's sake.

The next day, Grandad came home from the hospital. He looked weaker already – and he had a tube inserted in his throat which had to be attached to a machine every night, in order to clear the congestion from his lungs and to help him to breathe. The good news was that he could still walk. Every morning though, the nurse had to wash him and help him to dress, before he could join us in the sun lounge for breakfast. He liked to start the day by filling out his crossword puzzle.

I popped over each day to join Grandad for morning coffee. Occasionally the two of us took a walk in his back garden with the birds singing – although the nurse had to come too, to make sure that he did not fall. He took to wearing a scarf around his neck, to disguise the tube and prevent infection from entering his body. He managed to remain cheerful though – he was a very brave man. But the cancer was taking its toll, and soon he could not even speak – the cancer had spread to his voice box.

He had to communicate with pen and paper, but found this a slow and frustrating process. Rich had a brainwave one day. We went to Roberts Toy Shop together to buy supplies, and we took them straight over to Grandad. Grandad was puzzled when Rich showed him the small pads. 'They work like this,' Rich explained. 'You write here, then you pull out the side and push it back in again, and the writing disappears. Then you can use them again. No pens getting lost, or running out of ink – and an endless supply of paper!'

Grandad began to write on one of the pads, and we had to laugh when we saw what he had written. 'You're learning from your Grandad. About time too. Well done lads!'

He was a lot happier after that – he could communicate much more easily now. He had constant company, which he enjoyed. Mum, Dad and I saw him every day, and so did some of his other relatives and friends. His good friend Molly, who we called 'Auntie Molly' (we were friends with her family too) stayed over at the house with him regularly. My sister Julie visited too – she lived in Somerset, but she came to see Grandad often. He was stable and being well looked after, and although he was often in pain he never complained.

We had a lot of thunderstorms that year – I enjoyed these, I liked to watch them. Weather was a hobby for me – I would study the cloud formations, and liked watching programmes on TV about storms, especially tornadoes.

On the 16th October, the day before my birthday, I was invited to my friend's birthday party in Bournemouth. As I drove there, I sensed something strange in the air – the trees were unusually still. It was getting dark, but the temperature was rising, and the air was humid. I felt vaguely uneasy.

This feeling persisted when I arrived at the party, where all my friends were enjoying themselves without a care in the world. I kept looking at the sky – I sensed that something was not right, although I couldn't put my finger on what was wrong. I felt as if something heavy was bearing down from above, and something big was about to happen.

Because of the warm weather, the party was in the garden. There was a barbecue, and tables and chairs laid out on the patio. There were loads of people drinking and dancing. My friend Lynne came over and asked if I wanted to dance. When I said no, she looked at me in concern. 'What's wrong?' she asked. 'Are you in pain?'

'Not really,' I said. 'I just feel a bit odd. It's very hot, isn't it?'

'It certainly is for October,' she said.

Max came over then – he was the host of the party. He asked if I would like some birthday cake, and then he too enquired what was the matter.

'Look at the trees in your garden,' I said. 'They're stock still, and the temperature is still going up. I don't like this at all'. I think my friends thought it was a bit odd that I was so concerned about the weather, but just then Max's Mum came out of the house looking worried.

Max's Mum said that she'd been watching the weather forecast, and that Michael Fish had forecast a massive storm. However, he'd assured viewers that the full force of the storm would pass through the English Channel.

'That explains it,' I said.

'Explains what?' asked my friend's Mum.

'Why the trees are so still,' I said. 'It's the sign of a storm coming in. I have a feeling that the storm may not pass us by, after all'.

'Don't you worry about it,' she said. 'Just relax now and enjoy the party'.

I took her advice, and spent the next hour talking and dancing with the others. However, soon the wind blew up, and Max's Mum said she thought it would be best if everybody went home as soon as possible. I rang my Mum to say that I was on my way back, and she asked me to hurry home, and that my Dad would be waiting up.

As I drove home the wind was so strong that I could hardly steer straight. I had to take various diversions to get back, because many trees had crashed down and were lying across the roads, and across houses and cars too. Emergency service vehicles were racing everywhere. It was chaos. I eventually managed to reach Christchurch, where I was stopped by the police. 'Where are you going, son?' asked the policeman.

'Purewell,' I told him.

'That's fine, carry on,' he said. 'If you had been going to Highcliffe I would have had to stop you – the road in is closed. A block of flats has lost its roof'.

I managed to get home, although even after I had parked my car I had trouble getting into the house – the wind was lifting my car and bouncing it sideways, and the force of it made it hard to open my door. Eventually I used my feet to push my way out.

Dad had seen me drive up, and was waiting by the front door, which he opened just as I approached, and I managed to scramble inside. He put on the radio then, and we listened to the broadcast together. We heard about the many pensioners being rescued from the block of flats in Highcliffe that the policeman had just told me about.

There were many houses and cars destroyed by that storm – it was a major disaster along the South Coast. Many caravan parks and boats in Christchurch had been destroyed. The radio also announced that two firemen had been killed by a huge tree crashing on top of their engine in Highcliffe. Dad and I were really shocked to hear this.

The next morning was a clear, cold day. The sun was shining in a fresh blue sky, as if it was a new world. It was hard to believe that such chaos had reigned the night before.

'I'm off to Ashtree House,' I announced to my Dad. 'I want to open my birthday cards with Mum and Grandad'.

'I'll be over in a minute to join you,' Dad said.

Luckily my car was okay, but many others in the neighbourhood were severely damaged. Driving the short distance to Ashtree House was like being in a war zone, driving through the aftermath of a battle.

Grandad was pleased to see me. 'Happy Birthday, son,' he wrote on one of his pads. Then Uncle Matt came in, with the news that some of the stables were badly damaged. Dad arrived then. He was distraught. He told us all that he'd heard that Uncle David was one of the local firemen who had been killed in the storm last night. Grandad got out of his chair and went over to my

Mum, giving her a big hug. All of us cried then, thinking of Uncle David and his wife Auntie Joyce, who had been Mum and Dad's best friends. They had served in the fire brigade together in the sixties.

I knew the couple well – they had come to visit me in Great Ormond Street Hospital when I was young, and I was very fond of them. Dad rang Julie then, to tell her the news, and she was extremely upset too. Every year on my birthday I remember Uncle David, and his colleague Graham White, who died on the night of the great storm. I always take a few minutes to think about them, and of how they gave their lives to save others.

Grandad's health was deteriorating. He had to stay in the Macmillan Unit at Christchurch Hospital each night, although he was allowed home during the day. He was always cheerful, and courteous to the nurses who cared for him.

In November, Grandad invited all his friends and family to celebrate his eightieth birthday at Ashtree House. Rich and I did the disco, playing Grandad's favourite, Mantovani, as well as James Last's party hits. Near the end of the night Grandad wrote on one of his pads and showed it to us, 'Don't forget to end the show with God Save the Queen – or else!'

To finish the evening, he cut his birthday cake, and one of his friends read out a speech that he had written. 'I am very sorry,' it read, 'To have caused you all so much fuss and bother recently. I know time is running out for me. But I would like to ask you all to always stick together. Friends and family are the really important thing in this life!' We all applauded Grandad then – he was a very inspirational man.

1988 started with a huge shock for the whole family – my Uncle Matt suddenly died, and we were all devastated. I have great memories of my Uncle and I still cherish them all - how he made me a special trolley so I could see the Christchurch Regatta, how he bought me a USA spider bike, and later a motorbike. Matt loomed large in my life – he had got me the job at the goat farm, and even helped me sell red worms from a dung heap to the local fishing tackle shop.

I would also never forget our eventful trip to Scotland to pick up the horses. That was really something. But now I had to learn to live with those memories, and without Matt, and that was almost unbearably sad. My sister Julie came up to Christchurch to stay at Ashtree House, and help with the riding business. It was impossible to plan for the future though – nobody knew how long Grandad had left to live, and the inescapable facts of his illness and of Matt's death overshadowed all our lives.

By February it was clear that Grandad was drifting away. He had to stay full-time at the Macmillan Unit now, cared for around the clock by nursing staff. One evening I stayed with him alone for several hours. I held his hand and gazed at him while he slept. At one point he opened his eyes and looked at me, and I squeezed his hand lightly so that he knew I was nearby. He shut his eyes again. I kissed his hand then and said, 'Goodbye Grandad. Say hello to Nanny and Uncle Matt for me'.

The next day Grandad passed away. Ashtree Riding School was closed, and by the end of the year it was sold with its nine acres of land, and Ashtree House was sold separately, to a well-known local family. I knew this was necessary, but it still made me sad – I felt as though I had lost my true home.

Chapter Twenty-Three
Hair Today, and Gone Tomorrow

In October I had a big party for my 30th birthday, at the Royal Exeter Hotel in Bournemouth. Mr Jones, the manager, had let us have the party at a discounted price. I must have enjoyed the party, I suppose, although I was so cut up after Grandad's death that really I felt as though I was just sleepwalking throughout most of that year. The time passed in a blur – I have no idea what else happened in 1988.

So, before I knew it, 1989 had arrived. My signwriting business was still going strong, although I had to work at home now, in our garage, designing the signs for my customers. After a while I got depressed being stuck in there, so I decided to keep the garage door open while I worked, despite the cold weather. As Spring came in, and the weather warmed up, I sometimes moved out onto the driveway with my work.

Mum and Dad were members of the New Forest District Association Camping Club of Great Britain and Ireland. This was a nice hobby for them – most weekends they went off to the countryside, to caravan meetings with other club members. It was a lot more salubrious than 'Carry on Camping' – or so they assured me!

One day around April I was commissioned by the Camping Club to draw and paint sixty children's book characters – cartoons from The Jungle Book and so on – to be displayed in a huge Marquee, for the South West Region Summer Meet. I was also asked to design a display for the stage with the letters 'SWR' in huge print. The job took me several months in total, but I gained a sense of satisfaction from seeing my work on display.

Mum and Dad went on holiday for a week, and since I was at a loose end I decided to ring my friend Janette, to ask her if she would dye my long hair light blond. She came around straight away, but then looked doubtfully at me. 'I really need to take a sample of your hair to test, Anton, before I put any colour on it,' she said.

I told her not to worry, and that I was sure it would be fine, and she reluctantly agreed to go ahead. 'Don't blame me if it goes pear-shaped, though,' she insisted.

So she did the job, and it turned out very well indeed – I looked like Prince Charming! The next morning, though, I looked in the mirror when I woke up and gasped in shock – my lovely new long blond tresses had turned a bright lime green colour overnight! I looked like one of the Munchkins out of the Wizard of Oz. I was panicking. I had no idea what to do – I didn't want to call Janette, because after all she had warned me of what might happen.

Eventually I remembered Phil, one of my customers who owned a hair salon in Bournemouth. I rang him immediately and told him that my hair was green. 'Keep calm, Anton,' he said, 'I'll come over straight away'.

Phil was at my house within half an hour, and when he saw me he laughed his head off. He looked at my hair closely, and said that it still had chemicals in it, and then he washed it for me, and spent hours trying to sort it out. Eventually he sighed in despair. 'There's really not a lot I can do to make this better,' he said.

'I am so embarrassed,' I told him. 'I can't go out like this. I will just have to stay at home for ever'.

He laughed again. 'Don't give up,' he told me. 'If you don't mind me using your phone, I'll call a friend who may be able to help'.

He had a chat with his friend Terry, who agreed to give it a go, and Phil directed me to his shop. As soon as I got there, Terry greeted me effusively. 'Hello, Anton darling! So pleased to meet you! Now if you sit down and wait there, Mandy will bring you a cup of tea, and I'll be back in just a jiffy!'

Terry was back in minutes, trailing a trolley full of hair stuff. 'Now,' he said, 'Take your hat off, darling, and let's have a good look at you!'

'Wow,' he said when he saw my hair.

'Can you get me out of this mess?' I asked desperately.

'Er, kind of,' he replied. 'I'll have to cut off all your hair though, give you a short back and sides. Then we'll shampoo it off and run a few highlights through, and that should do the trick. You'll be here for the rest of the day though'.

'How much will it cost?' I wondered.

'We'll talk about that later,' he said. 'Just trust me, sweetie'.

Soon Terry was ready to begin. 'Are you ready for the big snip, then?' he asked.

'Yes and no,' I said nervously. Really I was dismayed to think that my long hair was going to be cut short.

'Well, the best thing for you to do is close your eyes,' said Terry. 'I'll tell you when to open them again'.

So I closed my eyes tightly and sat still for what seemed like an extremely long time, listening to the sharp snipping of his scissors. Terry was like a car mechanic, working fast and efficiently on my hair. When he eventually said that I could open my eyes I was sorry to see my hair so short, although I had to admit that he had given me a very good cut.

Next for the highlights. Terry mixed various chemicals to make a white paste, which smelt horrid, and then brushed sections of my short green hair with the mixture, rolling it up with cotton wool, and covering it with strips of what looked like cling film. He certainly seemed to know what he was doing.

I then had to sit under a hair dryer, next to two old ladies reading magazines. It was very noisy under there, although there was an interlude for a while when there was a power failure. I was there for ages, waiting for the power to come back on. When I caught sight of my reflection in a large mirror. I looked like a small spaceman ready for take-off, sitting under that huge hair dryer!

Eventually, Terry declared my hair ready to be washed and styled, and finally my ordeal was over. Everyone said that my hair really suited me short, although I missed my long hair already. The highlights looked good though, and at least I no longer needed to feel embarrassed to venture out in public.

I thanked him profusely. 'That's fine,' he replied. 'But

remember, don't let anyone turn you into a Munchkin again. Bye now, angel!'

Mum rang that evening, to ask what I'd been up to. 'Not much,' I said. 'I've been chilling out in the garden most of the time. And I did a short cut'. I went straight to bed after that, exhausted from my busy day, full of highlights (get it?)!

In October that year I was asked to help a couple whose teenage daughter had been in a car accident, and had ended up with one leg shorter than the other. She was refusing to go back to school, because she was worried that she would be laughed at, wearing a built-up shoe.

I met the girl, and spoke with her. I told her that I understood her fears, because I had felt the same about my first pair of special shoes. I showed her my shoes, and she was shocked – her shoe was not nearly as high, and I think that made her realise that her problems were not as serious as she had thought. She did go back to school, to her parents' relief, and I heard that not long after she went back to hospital and had a successful operation to lengthen her leg – so that story had a happy ending.

I was still doing discos, and I had an arrangement with the owner of a local pub, the Castle Tavern, to DJ there every weekend. I was having trouble breathing though, and had developed pains in my chest, especially on the evenings when I did the discos. Eventually I took myself to see the GP.

He checked my blood pressure and chest. 'You have a very bad chest infection,' he said, 'But your blood pressure is normal, and you have no problems with your heart as far as I can tell'.

'I have never felt this ill before,' I told him. 'Do you think I am developing asthma?'

'Hmm...' he said. 'Do you smoke?'

'Not personally,' I said. 'But the pubs where I do my discos are very smoky, and I inhale a lot of it. After the discos are over my clothes stink of smoke'.

'I am sorry to say that your disco days are over, Mr Evans,' he said, looking at me very seriously. 'That's what's causing your chest problems, and they won't go away until you stop'.

I took the doctor's advice regretfully, and sold all my disco equipment and my collection of 1000-plus records. I was sorry to have to do this, but I knew that it was more important to keep myself healthy.

I was given a present around that time, by an old college friend, Declan, who turned up to visit me unexpectedly. The gift he gave me was an album called 'Happy Talk' by someone called 'Captain Sensible' who I had never heard of before. Declan said he was giving it to me to cheer me up, because he knew the last year had been tough for me. 'Thanks,' I said, 'I'll play it to myself at Christmas time'.

'How are you keeping, anyway?' I asked my friend. 'I haven't seen you for ages'.

'Oh, I'm fine,' he replied. 'I have a new home, near the River Hamble. In fact, I have a project there that you might be able to help me with. I should be ready to get started by April, if you want to come over and see me then'.

'I'll look forward to it,' I said. 'It sounds very exciting'.

On Christmas Eve I did listen to that record. It did cheer me up too – because I dressed up as Captain Sensible and treated myself to a whole bottle of my favourite tipple, Martini Asti. 'Merry Christmas, everyone!' I declared, perhaps a trifle incoherently. It was the end of the Eighties!

In the New Year I was approached by three business partners to help with their new venture – they had bought the two lodges at the entrance to Highcliffe Castle, originally the main gatehouses, and they wanted to turn these into a restaurant.

The restaurant was to be called the Lord Bute, and the businessmen asked me to design a logo and some signs for it.

I racked my brains for this project, and eventually (after many hours at the drawing board, and plenty of cups of tea to keep me fuelled) I came up with a design. I then created two main signs for the entrance to the lodges, and many other signs for the restaurant itself. I even had to design menu covers printed in gold and black lettering.

The restaurant, when it opened, was very impressive. There were a wide range of dishes to choose from, and the catering was always top quality. The three partners became good friends of mine. Two of them were twin brothers, and they were very cool-looking. They were great fun to be around – they loved tap dancing and entertaining and they took part in the Black and White Minstrel Show in Bournemouth one year, inviting Mum and I to watch. I worked on that too, helping the company with their mobile wardrobe.

The time soon came to visit my friend Declan at his house in Hamble, on the Solent. I was really impressed with the huge house, and the garden, which Declan told me was eight acres long. However, he said he found it rather a lonely place, and wondered if I could help him come up with any ideas to use it productively. He said he wanted to set up some sort of activity in the garden, preferably one that would involve him mingling with other people.

'I need to take some photographs of the house,' I told him. 'But I'm afraid my legs won't manage the whole length of your garden'.

'I've got just the thing,' my friend replied. 'You can travel on my four wheel lawn mower'.

So we traversed the garden together, chatting and taking pictures. His housekeeper then made us lunch, which we ate in the conservatory of his wonderful house. After a while, Declan looked at me. 'Have you thought of something?' he asked. 'I can see you smiling'.

'I have had an amazing idea,' I said. 'You're going to need a landscape gardener, though, and an architectural designer who can survey your garden. I think you should build two large bowling greens on your land, and incorporate an octagonal pavilion to sell refreshments'.

I then expanded on my plan while Declan listened carefully. I suggested that he should have one green for the local bowling club, and another for the disabled, and that he should also make provision for car parking.

My friend was absolutely delighted with my idea. We chatted it through and when it was time for me to leave, he got out his cheque book and asked how much I wanted for my help.

'You don't need to pay me anything,' I said. 'Just hang on and see if you get planning permission. If not, you can take me out for a drink at the Jolly Sailor'.

1990 was another World Cup year. I hoped that Brazil would come through, but I had a bad feeling about it – which turned out to be right when Brazil lost to Argentina in the quarter final. I didn't lose faith in Brazil though – I still believe they are the best international team of all time!

That year I turned thirty-two, and I started my birthday chilling out, listening to music. After a while I got bored though, and headed up to Bournemouth, to browse Eddie Moors, my favourite music shop. I noticed they were selling new Yamaha keyboards, and started to play one, to see how it sounded. I got carried away playing lots of tunes, and when I stopped I heard applause breaking out in the shop behind me. I went red as a beetroot – I hate playing in public and hadn't realised anybody was listening!

Christmas was quiet that year, without Grandad and because a lot of members of our extended family had moved away. Mum, Dad and I had a simple celebration with Julie and her family. I was sad, because I missed my Grandad. But I knew that nobody could turn the clock back – and we still had our memories. At one o'clock sharp, Dad raised his glass in a toast and gave a short speech, 'To our family and friends' The one o'clock toast is a tradition that we still carry out today.

In 1991 my business slowed, because the United Kingdom was entering another deep recession. Thousands were losing their jobs each day – it was a very dispiriting time. There was also a diplomatic crisis when the United Kingdom expelled all Iraqi diplomats from the country. This was due to Iraq's invasion of Kuwait five months earlier. Matters quickly escalated when oil prices rose sharply. Before long, the Gulf War began, with the Royal Air Force joining Allied aircraft, beginning bombing raids in Iraq.

Things were so bad that I was worried that my business might go under, so at the end of the year I recruited a friend to help me. The plan was that he would work for me as a sales representative, on a commission only basis, and hopefully drum up some work for me.

Apart from the fact that I had no new work coming in, many of my current customers had not paid me what they owed, so I had serious cash flow problems. Even when I did get paid it was often delayed, which caused difficulties because my own workers and creditors were also awaiting payment.

I went to see my bank manager, but he refused to give me an overdraft. Luckily Mum came to my rescue, giving me a loan and helping me to organise my bookkeeping, so I managed to stay afloat, thank goodness.

Politics were coming to the fore again – there was due to be a general election on the 9th April, 1992. I saw the party political broadcasts on TV – John Major for the Tories, and Neil Kinnock for Labour. Kinnock promised a strong economic recovery if he was voted in – and I thought, 'Yeah, yeah. I've heard it all before!' Politics seemed to work like that, on a cycle – recession, recovery, recession – regardless of what the different parties or their leaders said or did. If anyone asked me my opinion about the upcoming election, I always told them that I would be voting for Lord Sutch and the Monster Raving Loony Party!

I had other things to think about anyway – the survival of my business was top of the list. My friend, now my sales rep, was working hard on my behalf, but was having trouble finding me work because there was so much competition. Many signwriters who had lost their jobs in the recession were starting up their own small businesses, so I had to be very competitive on price, which did not leave much margin for profit.

One day, to my delight, my rep arrived with good news. He had found me some work at the Avon Tyrell Youth Centre in the New Forest. I went over there immediately, and introduced myself to the manager, who asked me to design a new entrance sign. I suggested the Youth Centre Logo, and a colour illustration of the main house, and he was very pleased with that.

I was also asked to make emergency signs for fire exits, fire buckets and so on. I made a 999 sign for the phone, but the manager asked me to change it to 666, for their on-site phone boxes. The idea was that when someone called 666 it would alert the staff in the main house, who would decide whether the emergency services needed to be involved.

One morning I arrived early at the Youth Centre to find a mother panicking. She had tried to call 999 on one of the Avon Tyrell phones, but had not been connected to the emergency services. Her young son was frantic with distress – he had been bitten by an adder, and its fangs were still embedded in his thumb. The snake was hanging on for dear life, and I could see its poison running up the long vein in his arm.

I told the mother to call 666, and I used my handkerchief as a tourniquet, to stop the poison riding any further up the boy's arm, while I endeavoured to keep him calm. By the time the ambulance arrived the snake had let go of the boy's thumb. He was rushed to Southampton Hospital, where he made a complete recovery. Later in the day the Youth Centre manager and the boy's mother both praised me for my quick thinking. I spent many more weeks at Avon Tyrell and I loved the surroundings. I was sorry when all the signs were finished and my time there was over.

I had a quiet birthday at home that year – I was now thirty-four years old. At the end of October, I was invited to a Halloween party. I did not really want to go but my friend persuaded me, saying that I was always working, and I needed to get out and socialise more. I went as 'A Little Devil' and it turned out to be great fun.

In December, I had requests from numerous families, asking me to paint Disney characters for their disabled children. Somehow I had become known for doing this, and I enjoyed the work (I never took payment for it, of course). However, there were copyright issues, so this year I came up with a plan – I would design my own cartoon characters, to give as future Christmas gifts. I resolved to start in the New Year.

Mum, Dad and I had a good Christmas – we were cushioned from the worst effects of the recession, as my Dad still had plenty of plumbing work. However, I was well aware that all around the country other families were suffering, and that all the lost jobs meant less money to be spent in the festive season. I was very grateful still to be living in the midst of plenty, when so many others were forced to go without.

The start of the year was slow for me though – unemployment rates were rising fast, and there was not much money about. I managed to find some small pieces of work to keep busy though. Meanwhile, my sales rep and I designed a new Purewell Signwriters brochure and a small portfolio of coloured photos to show all the signs I had recently made, with a price list attached.

My rep decided to go out on the road to tout for business. His plan was to concentrate on selling my signwriting services to garden centres, hotels and tea rooms in Hampshire. I was pleased that he was being so proactive, but also a bit nervous – petrol did not come cheap and he would be out a lot. I hoped he would find some work soon.

I waited by the phone for the next week, hoping that a call for some work would come in. At the weekend I finally allowed myself to relax, and it was then, while I was watching television, that my Mum said there was a gentleman on the phone asking about new signs.

It was the owner of the Everton Water Garden Centre near Lymington, and he had a big order for me. I drove out immediately and really liked the place, which had a large shop, and many ponds dotted with water lilies and filled with enormous fish. The owner, who was a very congenial man, lived in a picturesque cottage on site.

I worked at the Water Garden Centre for a month. I made two large signs for the entrance, engraved with the name of the Centre, and instructed Todd, my sign-writer, to illustrate them with a cartoon of a frog leaping out of a pond between some bulrushes. The owner and I became firm friends.

The rep soon came up with another job for me – designing and printing more than 200 jam pot labels for the Manor Tea Rooms in Burley. This was a nice little job, although a bit fiddly!

I woke up one morning in so much pain from my hips and knees that I could not get out of bed. I screamed for my parents, who both came running to my side. Mum treated me with a painkilling spray, and when it had no effect she called the GP. He examined me and then spoke to me sternly.

'Mr Evans,' said the doctor, 'You are seriously over-doing things, and you have made yourself unwell. If you don't slow down immediately matters will worsen – your spine and rib cage could be affected and your mobility will suffer. Do you understand what I am saying?'

'I do, Doctor,' I replied, 'But I have a lot of work coming in at the moment, and I don't want to let my customers down'.

'You have not listened to a word I have said, have you?' he replied. 'You need to have two weeks' total rest, effective from today. Have you been riding your bike regularly, as I instructed you?'

'Erm, no,' I admitted. 'I keep forgetting'.

The doctor said that when my two weeks of enforced rest were up, I should start riding my bike daily around the local area. He said I needed to exercise my hips and knees in this way, to grind off the arthritis. He also referred me to the specialist at Southampton Hospital for further investigations.

The hospital appointment soon came through. I had X-rays on practically every bone in my body. Finally, the specialist examined me, and said that he had some bad news. 'I am sorry to tell you,' he announced, 'That every one of your joints is eighty per cent arthritic. Only your neck is currently free of the affliction. Your lifestyle and heavy workload are clearly not doing you any good whatsoever'.

'Are you saying I have to give up work?' I asked.

'By all means keep your business going,' he replied. 'But your disability is worsening and it would make sense to delegate your workload to others'.

Soon afterwards I spoke to Tod, who agreed to help more with my work. The rep was bringing in regular work now, and turnover increased. To keep busy I got on with the cartoon designs that I had been planning. The cartoons were called 'Antro's Cartoons Worldwide' and had a logo of a small music conductor.

I created and drew The Friendly Environment Gang, comprising five characters – Molezart the Mole, Archey the Oak Tree, Barny the Owl, Freddy the Fox and Franky the Frog. I hand painted ten copies of each character onto large A1 posters, and sent a set of five posters to ten children's hospitals all over the world.

By the start of 1994, although the recession was still going strong, and the economics of the country were not generally good, my business seemed to be getting back on track. I had only small amounts of work coming in, because people seemed to be holding on to their money, but it was enough to keep me going.

Now I designed a second set of posters to be sent to children's hospitals. This time, I created fruit characters – Percy the Pear, Oscar the Orange, Alfred the Apple, Sir Grape the Grape and Viola the Banana. I painted ten copies of each, just as I had for the Friendly Environment Gang, but this time instead of sending the posters worldwide, I sent them to children's hospitals within Europe. I kept the copyright for my characters again.

I had another project on – I painted a copy of a Lion King picture, which I took from a magazine. I was really pleased with it, although of course I could not sell it because of copyright issues. Later the same day, a lady walked past my garage, where I was painting with the door open as usual. 'You are always painting,' she said. 'I see you every time I walk past. You remind me of Demis Roussos. Have you heard of him?'

'Erm, no,' I told her.

'He's a very famous Spanish singer,' she said. 'I saw him at a concert in London, and he has the most amazing voice'.

Well, I thought to myself, he is not Spanish at all, he is half Greek and half Egyptian. I am not quite sure why I claimed not to know who Demis Roussos was – I think it was because the lady seemed to be quite a chatterbox and I was afraid that I would be caught in conversation for the rest of the day!

In May of 1994, the Channel Tunnel was officially opened. I found the prospect of travelling by train between England and France very exciting. It gave me hope that perhaps I was one step nearer to visiting Paris, which had been my dream for some time. I saw that city as being a magical place, filled with history, architecture and wonderful works of art. Maybe one day I would see it for myself!

In June, the World Cup took place in the USA. This time, I felt in my bones that Brazil were going to win – and they did it! I was beside myself with happiness. That year I was thirty-six, and as a gift to myself I rented a Toshiba TV and a Mitsubishi video recorder for my bedroom, because I had decided that I wanted to be more independent at home.

Chapter Twenty-Four
The Recession Ends

Soon it was 1995, and the United Kingdom was slowly coming out of the recession at last. Unemployment was falling – hurrah for that, I thought, because even though I had my own business now I knew how it felt to be out of work, and I wouldn't wish it on anybody.

I had a lot of new customers for my signwriting business, and I felt happy and secure. Then I went down with a flu virus, which not only affected my legs, arms and ribs but also gave me terrible headaches. I had very bad mouth ulcers, that made it difficult and painful to swallow. Mum called the doctor out, and he diagnosed tonsilitis. My condition worsened, and soon I was coughing up blood. I slept in the front room because I was too weak to manage the stairs. I could hardly manage to eat and I developed such a high temperature that I became delirious and Mum had to call the doctor out again.

One evening there was a flash in the back of my left eye, and I went blind. It only lasted for a few minutes, but during that time I panicked and managed to knock my radio onto the ground, where it smashed into bits. I lost weight, and became so weak that I could not stand. I could not stop coughing, day and night. The doctor was called yet again, and pumped me with antibiotics, but nothing seemed to help. It was almost two months before I recovered from the flu, but it left me so weak and sickly that I could still not eat proper food. This time, the doctor made me an appointment to see the specialist at Bournemouth Hospital.

To my surprise, the specialist asked whether I had kissed

any girls recently. 'I don't have a girlfriend,' I told him. 'But I did kiss my friend's wife to wish her Happy Birthday, a while ago. She was a bit poorly at the time. Is there a connection, then?'

'There could be,' replied the doctor. 'You have glandular fever, which is sometimes referred to as the Kissing Disease, because it can be caught that way. Unfortunately, symptoms can hang about for a while – it could be a year before you are fully well again'.

I was horrified to hear this, but there was nothing I could do. I did slowly recover, and managed to struggle on with some work – I remember signwriting and illustrating an open air ice cream parlour with wheels, something I had to rush to complete before the Easter holidays.

Around that time I went to visit my Nanny Evans, who was in failing health at a nursing home in Bournemouth. I stayed with her for an hour, although she kept drifting off into sleep. She died just a few days later, on Easter Sunday, and we were all heartbroken. The funeral was attended by many of her family and friends. I attended the church service, which was very short, but I could not go to the cemetery because I felt too unwell. I drove there a week later instead, to put flowers on her grave.

It was a grey day, as miserable outside as I felt inside. I sat on a bench near Nanny's grave, and I couldn't stop crying. Then a man appeared – he looked like an Orthodox Jew, with a long black coat and hat. He sat next to me. 'What a nice car you have,' he said (my car was parked nearby). 'We need the sun to come out, to make everybody warm and happy'.

Just as I turned to reply, he had vanished! He was nowhere to be seen, which was strange, because there was no place for him to have gone. It was very mysterious. I am not a religious person, but that encounter felt mystic, and I puzzled over it for some time.

One evening, at home alone, I decided to watch an Indian film which was on the TV. It was due to start at nine o'clock and I made myself comfortable in advance, finding the biscuit tin that Mum always hid from me, and taking a large packet of chocolate Digestives from it. I poured myself a large glass of Martini and lemonade to wash them down with.

The film was absolutely fantastic! It was a Bollywood production, a romantic comedy musical, and I was spellbound! After that I began to watch more Bollywood films, loving the music, dancing, and costumes and the romantic and funny story lines.

I also saw a wonderful singer on television around that time – she was called Hasna and was from Morocco. She sang 'Far Away' with Demis Roussos! I loved foreign music, and learned to speak the basics of Arabic, Greek and French. I learned to play some of this music on my electronic keyboard, including a French song called Quand Je T'Aime (When I Love You) by Demis Roussos.

My friends became worried, asking me whether I was anti-British, because I seemed to prefer foreign music and cinema! I said no, that I was proud to be British, but that I liked the culture of other countries too.

That year I turned thirty-seven. On my birthday I went

out with a friend to Stanpit Marsh, to help fly his stunt kite. This had cost him more than four hundred pounds, and was a wonderful 'toy' – made from proper sail material. He flew it on two strings, and it often landed in the water, but he managed to pull it back up. However, the final time he landed it in the water it became tangled up in the propeller of a speedboat, and nearly caused a serious accident! We had to slink off, tails between our legs!

There was another near miss later that year, on Fireworks Night, the 5th November. I had been invited to a party at a friend's house in Sopley, and I took along the biggest and most expensive rocket I could afford. However, when the rocket was lit, it misfired, falling over and exploding almost horizontally to the ground. We all dived for cover, and fortunately we escaped harm, as the rocket flew through the gap between two parked cars, hitting a water trough and finally exploding harmlessly into a bush.

In 1996, my business seemed to be getting back on track. I now asked for payment up front from my customers. I was not just sign-writing – I had also decided to design my own children's books, using the characters from the Friendly Environment Gang and the Friendly Fruit Gang.

I joined forces with my friend's sister, who wrote poems to accompany my illustrations. She did an excellent job. Then I designed another set of characters – the Friendly Veg Gang. This set comprised Caracca the Carrot, Pierre the Pea, Cabio the Cabbage, Patio the Potato and Ollie the Onion. My friend wrote poems for all these characters too. I sent copies of my books to many publishers, and in return I received many rejection letters!

Meanwhile, I embarked on another project, drawing some of the sites around Christchurch to create a poster and tourist book of the area. I used my bike a lot to get out and about and draw my pictures – I knew it was important for my health to keep moving. I did all the illustrations in black and white. I sold one thousand copies of the posters, books and bookmarks in the local gift shops in just two months, and made a healthy profit.

I also became involved with a local football team. My friend's wife asked if I would be interested in supporting the Archer's Arrows – their son played for the team. I agreed to sponsor the team, and in return for buying their new football shirts I had my Purewell Signwriters logo printed on the front of them. Mr Archer and the team were very pleased, and I had my picture taken with them for the sports page of the Bournemouth Echo.

In March of 1998, I decided to take a trip to Disneyland, Paris, with my sister and two of my friends. I booked a coach trip with Leger Holidays, and borrowed a Red Cross wheelchair to take with me just in case. Mum was worried about me going on such a long journey, but Julie promised that she would take care of me.

At 8am on the designated day, we boarded our huge continental coach. I was quite nervous about the trip, but the friendly, jocular drivers helped me relax. The coach was only half-full, which was good, and we were in the front seats, so had a great view. We stopped twice on the way, at Brighton and Hastings, and finally arrived at Dover, ready to be ferried across to Calais in France.

Then our coach had to be checked by security, and we

also had to show our passports, before we could board the ferry. They checked everything – but not my built-up shoes, and it occurred to me that I could easily have hidden a bomb in those! I must have an innocent face...

There was a storm at sea, quite soon into our journey. I felt very sea-sick, and so did lots of other passengers. Fortunately I remembered the advice that I had been given on the Silver Jubilee cruise, to 'dance with the boat'. I did so, and it soon eased my discomfort – plenty of other passengers joined in too!

What should have been a one hour crossing became two, because of the storm. When we finally arrived at Calais, my first impression was that France was very flat! It was a long tiring journey, but I enjoyed the French music playing on the radio.

We finally arrived at 10pm. It was dark now, and the lights of our hotel – the Newport Bay - glowed ahead. It looked amazing. When I finally got to my room it was very posh, with its own TV and an en-suite bathroom. I had a double bed too, which felt like luxury. It was midnight, and I was exhausted, but before I went to sleep I made a video of myself, talking about the journey and my arrival at the hotel. This was a holiday I wanted to remember for a long time ahead!

I slept like a log, and in the morning went over to the big Disneyland theme park. It was magical there – not too busy because the children were all in school, but with a cracking atmosphere. I went on the underground pirate ride, which was great. I sat in a boat raft, and travelled through long dark tunnels, and at the end there was an unbelievably brilliant pirate display.

I was really enjoying it – but then suddenly the raft dropped down, and I was petrified. I was relieved when that ended – but then it happened again – another drop, and then a fast spin down a long twisted tunnel. I nearly wet myself with fear. I was so pleased to see daylight at the end of the ride, and when I got off that raft I was still shaking.

I saw Julie, 'How could you do this to me?' I asked.

'Blame Mum,' she laughed, 'She told me to get you on the pirate ride'.

In the gift shop I bought a French beret, which I have kept to this day. I felt a tap on my shoulder in the shop – and when I turned around it was a tall green monster! He had a good look at me, and then ran off as if he was scared – but I did manage to film him before he went. Lots of children were laughing at the spectacle – but whether they were laughing at him or me, I was not quite sure!

We ate at the hotel that evening – it was a lovely meal, and a very relaxing evening. My friends and I looked around the hotel lobby and gift shop. I reflected on the day – it had been such fun, I really liked the Disneyland castle and characters. I thought to myself what a force for good Disney was, joining all nationalities in the fun and magic, encouraging everyone to be happy, children and adults alike.

The next day we were off early to visit the city of Paris. I was sad to leave Disneyland, but very excited about seeing Paris at last. I videoed the whole journey! We stopped by the River Seine, in front of the Eiffel Tower, and it looked like a very romantic place to be. We saw the Arc de Triomphe, and many coffee shops, fashion shops, museums, parks and gardens, and artists, painting on the pavements. And of course the Eiffel Tower itself – an incredible impressive structure.

We had just two hours to look around Paris. Julie and my friends went to the Eiffel Tower, but I stopped to look at the paintings by the Seine. I met an artist selling beautiful oil paintings, who spoke good English and was very friendly. He had a friend, another artist, and we chatted about the recent tragedy in Paris, in which Princess Diana had died.

When I turned to say goodbye to the original artist I realised with a jolt that he had gone. He had vanished into thin air, and that was when I realised where I knew him from – he was the same man who I had seen near my Nanny Evans' grave. He had vanished that time too, and I was struck with wonder and puzzlement, just as before.

I bought some oil paintings, of a violin and a French cafe. Then it was time to meet my sister and my friends – my sister said that she had known I would buy paintings! We boarded the coach again, and toured some more sites. We even saw the place where Princess Diana's accident had happened. I could not stop thinking about the Jewish man and how strange it was to see him again, but I made myself bring my mind back to the present.

Paris is a wonderful city, and I promised myself that I would remember my trip forever. By the time I reached home I was very tired though, and in some pain. It was after midnight before I went to bed, and the next morning my Mum was very concerned at my condition.

'Are you in pain, son?' she asked.

'I am,' I admitted, 'But it was worth it, for such a wonderful holiday'.

Chapter Twenty-Five
Forty Years Young!

So – back to England, and to reality. It seemed a long time ago that I had first visited Great Ormond Street as a young boy, back in the Sixties. The specialist who broke the news of my disability to my parents had told them that I might never reach the age of forty. He said that as I got older my disability would worsen and my bones and breathing would be affected.

The specialist had been right in a way – my condition had deteriorated with age and I had a lot of pain in my joints, particularly when I moved. But I had no intention of giving up on life – I had a family, and a business to run! So I was looking forward to reaching my fortieth birthday and proving his dire prognosis wrong.

I wanted to celebrate this birthday, but although I racked my brains, I couldn't think what to do. In around June, Mum asked whether I would like to invite all my friends around for a birthday party. I said that I felt a bit old for that, but that she could decide.

'Why don't you sit down and write a list of what you would like for birthday presents?' she asked, but I got upset with her. I felt like she was treating me as a child.

'Can we not go on about it any more? I am buzzing off now, to get some peace!' I said. I slammed out of the front door and drove through the New Forest to Southampton Docks. I watched the big cargo ships coming in from the Solent, and slowly felt myself relax. Then, out of the blue, my mobile phone buzzed in my pocket. It made me jump – I had not yet got used to the new technology, which entailed everyone being constantly in touch by mobile phone.

It was one of the twins from the Lord Bute Restaurant. He asked me to meet him, and when I arrived at the Lord Bute both twins were waiting, smiling. They told me they knew that my 40th birthday was coming up, and asked whether I would like to have a special lunch in their restaurant, catering for forty friends and family.

I was so pleased with the offer, but said that I would need to ask my parents before I agreed. When I got home I was in a much better mood. Dad asked whether I had calmed down from that morning.

'I do feel happier,' I told him. 'I have just been offered a special price for a birthday lunch at the Lord Bute'.

'Your Dad and I have already booked it,' said my Mum. 'We were only teasing you this morning'.

'Well, I have changed my mind, in that case,' I said. 'I don't want a party now. I can't be bothered'.

They both looked horrified, and I burst out laughing. 'Only joking!' I said.

'You're grounded!' said Mum, 'Go to your room at once!'

'I think he's a bit old to be grounded now,' my Dad pointed out. 'He's almost forty, don't you know?' And we all laughed together.

Before my party, it was time for the FIFA World Cup again. This time the competition was held in France, and I was excited because Brazil were in the final, playing the French. The match was extremely tense, and unfortunately 'my' team did not win. I felt let down, but resigned myself to the fact that they'd have another crack at the Cup in four years' time.

On October 17th, the morning of my fortieth birthday, I woke up with tears in my eyes. I was thinking of Ashtree House and Grandad. I stared at the ceiling, lost in thought.

Mum tapped on my door, and came in. 'It's time to come downstairs soon,' she said. 'You might be getting something in the post!'

Ron, the postman, was a family friend, and he came into the kitchen with a huge bag of birthday cards for me. 'How does it feel being forty?' he asked.

'I suddenly feel very old,' I told him. Ron reassured me that forty was not old at all, and that I should see how I felt when I got to sixty, like him.

Julie arrived, and soon it was time to leave. To my surprise there was a chauffeur-driven vintage car waiting for me! I was to be driven to the restaurant in it, as a surprise present from my Dad. The car looked like one I had seen on TV in the 'Secret Service' series. However, secretly it reminded me of a sewing machine on wheels! It was also not terribly practical – there were no side windows, and it was a cold day. We slowly drove down the roads, and everyone we passed turned their heads to gaze at us, probably wondering what the special occasion was.

Finally we reached the Lord Bute, and I managed to climb out of the car with some difficulty. My nephew and niece had to hold me up between them until the circulation in my legs returned! Then they led me into the restaurant, where I was greeted by the most amazing sight. The place was decorated in the Brazilian colours, with green, white and blue balloons and flags everywhere. It was packed with my family and friends. It was great to see all my favourite people in one room.

The meal was very good, and I washed it down with Asti Martini. I was very contented. Then my nephew stood up and called out that he wanted to wish me a very Happy Birthday – and that he also wanted to say, 'Uncle Anton – This is Your Life!'

He held out a red book that had been compiled especially for me and he read out from it. It was wonderful, if a little embarrassing! Then I made a speech, thanking everyone for coming along and Mum and Dad in particular, for everything they'd done for me.

Later that afternoon, I got the biggest surprise of all. Bleeping through on my phone was a text message, from Ellie. 'Bonjour Anton,' it read, 'Happy 40th Birthday'.

I was shaking with surprise, overjoyed that I had heard from my ex-girlfriend for the first time in so many years. I realised that she must have got the number from her friend Charlie. But although I dearly wanted to see her again, I decided it would be wiser to let the past alone. So much had happened since we were young together. No, I decided, I would concentrate on my own life from now on.

In January of 1999, I was approached by two lads in their twenties, computer games designers. They wanted me to design and build a large castle for them, to use as a set for their warrior games. Computer technology was all new to me, but they said that they had faith in my ability to design what they wanted. They said they needed the castle in three months' time. I had no idea how to design a castle at first, or even what materials I should use, but after lots of failed attempts and plenty of discarded plans, I consulted some library books and knuckled down to the task.

I spent three months working on that castle, in the garage or on a table in the driveway. It was a fantastic creation, with many large and small towers, and it constantly attracted the attention of passers-by. I was very proud of it by the time I had finished – my nephew took a photo of me posing with it, like the King of the Castle! The lads were both very pleased with my work and paid me well.

I had another project to complete in December – I was asked to paint a big picture of Winnie the Pooh for a Christmas Grotto. I enjoyed this so much that I painted a big Christmas picture of Minnie and Mickey Mouse, outside the Paris Disneyland castle, which we fixed to the front of our house, above the garage door.

New Year's Eve that year marked the end of the Millennium, and I was happy to be invited to a friend's party in Sopley Park. I wore my Grandad Cook's Burma Star – a medal that he got when he was fighting the Japanese, in the Chindits. I decided that it was a good opportunity to commemorate him, and the others who fought alongside him for the freedom of our country. Without the valour and rigour of those men, the rest of us might not be here today.

And here we were – marking the end of a Millennium,

and about to embark on a new era!

At the beginning of the new Millennium, celebrations took place across the United Kingdom. The Millennium Dome was opened by the Queen, and I was very impressed with its design. It was located on the Greenwich Peninsula, in South-East London, close to the River Thames.

The Queen Mother celebrated her 100th Birthday, which was a real milestone for her and for the nation. She was my favourite Royal – I liked her because she was so chatty and such a great character. She reminded me of my Nanny Evans, in a lot of ways.

Wembley Stadium was closed in the year 2000, and I was sad to see the place go. I had fond memories of watching various football matches that had taken place there over the years, including the 1966 World Cup.

It was a harsh winter that year, with heavy snow and temperatures dropping as low as minus 13C. Luckily for us, we were able to stay warm and snug at home, safe in the knowledge that we had a plumber right on hand should our central heating choose to pack up!

I also had problems with my feet at that time. My surgical shoes were not suiting me – the leather was too thin, and they were most uncomfortable. It took many weeks to get an appointment with the consultant, and when I did see him he insisted that I needed to have short thick leather boots with a fixed zip. I told him that I thought the leather would rub on my ankles, but he would not listen. When the shoes were made, a month later, and I went back to Southampton Hospital to try them on, they were every bit as bad as I had anticipated.

The leather not only caused blisters on my ankles, they put my hips out of synch too, and I had trouble walking at all. I asked to see the consultant again, and was put back on the waiting list.

Around that time I employed a student to help me at work, because I was feeling unwell due to all the stress over my shoes. I was wearing my old shoes for the time being, but was worried that I would end up housebound if I could not get any suitable footwear.

I was pleased with the student – she was very clever with computer graphics, and a good worker. She even designed me a new flyer, advertising my boat signwriting skills. One day she drove me to the National Art Gallery in London, calling ahead to arrange use of a disabled parking space with the gallery, and to book the use of a wheelchair. We had a great day out, seeing many fantastic paintings at the Gallery, and other art at the Tate Modern, and even fitting in a trip to Madame Tussauds, where I met Pele and the Beatles (or at least their facsimiles!)

The only disappointment was at the end of the day, when we found a parking ticket on our car – we were parked in a disabled space but the car was one inch over the kerb, so we got booked. I was really cross about that, but luckily the National Gallery sorted it out.

In November, I paid to see the consultant privately about my shoes. He arranged for me to have new shoes, made with thicker leather, three times a year, which was the best result I could have hoped for.

I made another Christmas picture to go outside the house that year, with all the characters from Alice in

Wonderland. Dad fixed up lights to go around it. And of course, he heralded our Christmas dinner with a speech as usual, which Mum and I greatly appreciated.

Another year was over, and a new one began.

Early in 2002, I set up a new website for my Purewell Signwriters business, and this brought me many new customers. Now I just had to learn how to use the internet. I learned to use a computer keyboard, and started to send emails. I found that it was much quicker and easier for me to type on the keyboard than to write by hand. I also found it great to be able to get any information I needed, fast, through the Net. I did find some things particularly hard though – like learning the new technical signs and symbols on the keyboard.

Meanwhile, I heard from a local travel agent who had used one of my large Anton's Euro Castles to advertise holidays in 2001. They told me that the promotion had gone really well, and asked whether I would do them the honour of lending the castle again for the Queen's Golden Jubilee. I was really pleased to be able to help – it was nice to know that all my hard work was being put to good use.

Chapter Twenty-Six
A Visit to Tadworth Court

Back in the Eighties, Tadworth Court, the 'Country Branch of Great Ormond Street' had been taken over by a charity called The Children's Trust. I was keen to know more about the Trust, so I decided to visit Tadworth and see for myself how it was being used.

As soon as I arrived, I could see that the beautiful gardens and arched walkways remained the same, and that several new complexes had been built. Tadworth Court was still immaculate, which was heartening to see. One of the fundraising team members showed me round – I rode in a wheelchair. They talked to me about the Trust as we went.

The old canteen in the stable courtyard, where a nurse took me for tea back in 1973, was now the fundraising department offices. I was introduced to the fundraising team, who were working flat out on their phones and computers. Apparently, they needed to raise more than five million pounds each year, just to keep the Trust running, and so were constantly looking for sponsors to help support their fundraising events.

My friend videoed the visit, and I would treasure that video as a memento for many years to come. I was loath to leave the place – it was such a special place, and brought so many magical memories flooding back, and I was sad to say goodbye.

The Queen Mother died just a short time later, at the end of March. This was a very sad occasion too, although she had reached the grand old age of 101.
I watched the funeral broadcast live on the BBC, as

London came to a standstill, with thousands gathering to watch the procession. I cheered myself up with the thought that perhaps now my Nanny Evans and the Queen Mother were enjoying afternoon tea and a good gossip together!

The FIFA World Cup was hosted jointly by South Korea and Japan this year. I felt that Brazil would be okay this time, and really hoped that my instinct was correct. However, I was slightly torn, because of course England had qualified too, and were hoping to win for the second time. How, I wondered, could I be loyal to both teams?

This year was also the Queen's Golden Jubilee, and I was invited to a party to celebrate, at my friends' house in Bridport. They were having a barbecue. So I drove across Dorset on the appointed day. Before I left, I asked Mum to tape Brazil's first match against Turkey for me, so that I could watch it later.

When I got to my friends' house I could see that they had made a huge effort. There were loads of tables on the decking in their garden, all covered in food. There were flags everywhere. There were also loads of bottles of my favourite tipple, Martini, and my friends persuaded me that I would need to stay overnight, to do it all justice. I didn't take much persuading!

Many neighbours and friends soon arrived, and we all made merry. The Jubilee Celebrations were on the television. I decided to call my Mum, to tell her that I was staying the night, and while I was on the phone I couldn't resist asking how the match had gone.

'Brazil beat Turkey two goals to one,' she told me, and I whooped with joy.

The party was still going strong, and soon I was having problems standing up – for once though, this wasn't due to pain in my legs, but because I had spent most of the day imbibing Martini! I decided to have some food to counterbalance the alcohol, which worked, and I slept like a log that night.

I headed home bright and early in the morning, after thanking my friends. I was looking forward to getting back to the football, and was not disappointed. Brazil did really well, and were due to play England in the quarter-finals. My loyalty was divided, but Brazil were my team and I would not waver in my support for them. So, on June 21st, the day of the match, my Brazilian flag flew from my bedroom window, and my Mum's England flag flew alongside it from her room!

Christchurch was deserted that day - everyone was at home, watching the big match. David Beckham was a huge star by now, and he was playing for England – he really drew the crowds. I decided to drive out to Burley and listen to the match on the radio, in my secret location. I was very nervous about the outcome of this match, and I needed to be alone.

I looked out at the wonderful scenery of the New Forest, as I listened to the radio.   Twenty-three minutes in, Owen scored for England. The crowd went wild – but then to my surprise I realised that some of the cheering was coming from the car parked alongside mine. England football fans had invaded my secret location!

I was in shock, because my privacy had been disturbed, and because it looked as though England might win the game. Luckily though, Brazil scored just before half-time. 'Goal!' I shouted out in delight, and the passengers in the car next to mine glanced at me in disgust.

The second half of the game was full of action, and Beckham played well.   Eventually Brazil had a free kick though, and Ronaldinho lobbed it in past David Seaman from 42 yards, sending Brazil to the semi-finals. I was over the moon!

The couple from the next car got out, and came over to my window. 'Why are you not supporting your national team?' they asked angrily.

I answered in Portugese, and assuming then that I was Brazilian, they apologised, and I smiled graciously. I'd got away with that encounter, but wondered whether I would get lynched on my arrival home, from all the people who knew that I supported Brazil. Fortunately, nothing much was said – nobody took it personally, after all!

In the World Cup semi-final Brazil won one goal to nil against Turkey, with Ronaldo scoring on the forty-ninth minute. Hurrah – and now for the Final!

The final match of the cup was held in Yokohama Stadium in Japan, where Brazil played Germany.   I knew that the German side was strong and nobody knew how things would go – but to my delight Brazil won the World Cup for the fifth time! I was in tears of joy, and things got even better when many people in our street popped in to congratulate me. It was a good feeling.

The good feeling lasted – for my birthday that year (I was forty-four now) Mum organised a party for me at home, and made me a special birthday cake decorated in yellow, green, blue and white! I wore my Brazilian shirt with the same colours, and we all raised our glasses in a toast to the beautiful game, and to my own special team.

Christmas was wonderful too, with Mum's marvellous traditional lunch and wonderful Christmas pudding. At 1pm Dad did his speech as usual. 'Boo to Brazil!' he said, and we all chuckled at his joke. It was the end of a brilliant year.

The BBC news was big and scary at the start of 2003. Rumours abounded that Saddam Hussein was making chemical weapons of mass destruction, and killing his own people too, over in Iraq. Tony Blair's Labour government came to the conclusion that war on Iraq was the only way forward (despite two million people taking to the streets of London to protest against this, the largest demonstration in British history).

Meanwhile, in February, I received an urgent fax. It confused me at first, because it was written in French. Jasmine, a friend, translated it for me. 'This is very exciting!' she exclaimed as she looked it over. 'The customer is requesting that you create a small model castle to be sent to France for a carnival float in Nice. He says he needs delivery of the castle within two weeks!'

Jasmine explained to me why this was so exciting – she said that the Nice carnival is huge, second only to the Brazilian and Venetian ones. She then phoned the organiser for me. However, to our disappointment, we found that sadly, since faxing me, the chap had pulled out of the carnival parade due to lack of funding. So that was the end of that – over before it had begun!

On the 20th March, news came through that we were, as expected, officially at war with Iraq. We won that war, and now, of course, at the time of writing, we are at war with Afghanistan. It seems that we need to learn the lessons taught to us by history over and over again.

Anyway, that summer I wanted to build more castles, but I felt as though I had somehow run out of inspiration. So I drove to the New Forest, to my secret hideout in Burley. It was a beautiful day, and this was the best place I could think of to design my castles. I drew my designs on paper fixed to a clip board, immersed in my favourite occupation.

I managed to find a picnic table and set myself up with lunch. Nearby was a family enjoying a picnic of their own, and before long a boy approached to look at my drawing. 'Wow Mum!' he exclaimed. 'A castle!'

Suddenly, a large shadow loomed. It was a massive white bull, and I urged the little boy and his family to stay still and not to panic.

'Shh!' I told the boy. 'Hide under the table!'

The bull looked at me in a bad-tempered fashion, then stamped his hoof. I thought he was readying himself to charge. So I drew myself up to my full height and shouted at the creature, 'Boo!' To my relief, the bull retreated, and ran away. It could have gone either way – forwards or back, and I was so pleased that it chose the latter. The boy's family thanked me profusely, and I smiled modestly in return, and said, 'It was just one of those things. No worries! And,' I continued, 'You can come out from under that table now, young man!' and he crawled out and ran straight into the arms of his mother.

Chapter Twenty-Seven
Fame at Last!

In 2003, my birthday was an event to remember. That morning at the bank something quite wonderful happened. I could hear two children talking as I waited in the queue, 'There's Anton, the famous artist!' they said. 'He makes castles!'

I turned to say hello, but before I could speak, they asked for my autograph! I signed the back of a paying in slip for them, as I had no other paper to hand! When I got to the front of the queue there was more adulation – the cashier asked for my autograph too! 'Perhaps I am a famous artist,' I said to myself. (Or perhaps a 'Fartist'?!)

As December began, my thoughts turned to designing my Christmas scenery. I decided to paint a scene from Snow White, and whiled away several days engaged on this pleasant pastime – warm inside my garage studio, listening to Christmas carols on Classic FM.

Christmas was just around the corner, and then suddenly it was upon us. We had an idyllic day. In Dad's speech he remembered the British soldiers who had fallen in the Iraqi war, and we all bowed our heads in a gesture of silent respect to them all.

In the New Year, 2004, I had lots of phone calls from prospective customers, and several of them offered me work. In February I came up with a new business idea, making horse and pony name plaques for riding schools and equestrian centres. I designed leaflets to advertise my wares, and sent them out to riding schools all over the UK.

Several days after my mailshot, I had a call from Wild Woods Riding School in Surrey, very close to The Children's Trust. The owner of the school ordered twelve plaques over the phone, and we got talking about the Trust. He told me that the place used to belong to Great Ormond Street Hospital, and said that he'd owned a pig farm next to their land.

'I was a patient there in 1973,' I told him excitedly, 'And believe it or not, I visited your pig farm!' We agreed that it was quite a coincidence, and we chatted for some time.

The weather was getting warmer now, and I often worked outside my studio garage. Sometimes people would stop for a look and a chat - there were often traffic jams in our street!

One afternoon, out on a bike ride, I hit a pot hole and came off. Before I could even stand up, my phone rang. 'Where are you?' my Mum asked. 'I've been looking for you everywhere'.

I had cut my knee badly and when I got home my Mum fussed around me with antiseptic cream and plasters. It's not a bad thing having someone to look after you, I reflected as Mum cleaned me up. Even if they do still think you're a child! Mum had been eager to find me to pass on an urgent message from a photographic advertising agency. When I called them, the lady in charge said that she had an important job for me, from the Portman Building Society.

'We have a six foot handmade High Striker,' she said, 'Do you think you could paint it in vintage fairground colours, with numbers showing interest rates for savings accounts?'

'I might be able to,' I said, 'If I knew what a High Striker was'.

She laughed. 'It's a strength tester,' she told me, 'An attraction used at funfairs and carnivals. You hit a target using a hammer, and see if you can make the bell at the top of the tower ring'.

Now I understood what she meant, and I agreed to do the job. I enjoyed painting the High Striker, and the lady was delighted when I called her to say it was done. 'I didn't know you were disabled,' she said when she came to collect it. 'I must say, you have done a brilliant job on this. I love those castles too – they're beautiful'.

In June it was my Mum's 70th birthday. I made her a coffee cream birthday cake with musical candles. She cut the first slice and was about to tuck in when she started to laugh. 'Where has the bottom half of the cake gone?' she asked.

'I don't know what you mean,' I said.

'I can see there used to be more to this cake,' she said, 'And that means someone has been at it. And I think that someone was you. Am I right or am I right?'

'It is all to do with the government cuts,' I told her (but of course she had me bang to rights!).

'Thanks,' she said later. 'The top half of the cake tasted lovely'.

When it comes to birthday gifts, it's the thought that

counts, that's what I always say.

In July that year Dad turned seventy. He was hot and giddy on that day, and when the doctor came for a home visit, he said it was a touch of angina, and he instructed Dad to rest. My father had been diagnosed with angina some years before, but suddenly his blood pressure had become very high.

Dad was given a prescription for extra strong tablets to keep his blood pressure down, and after about a week he felt better again, and we all relaxed. However, one morning when I came down for breakfast, Dad was nowhere to be seen. Mum explained that he was tired, and that it was best to leave him to rest.

I went back upstairs after breakfast, and heard my father calling out for help, his voice croaking painfully. I rushed into his room and found him holding his hand to his chest. I called Mum, who dialled 999, and a paramedic soon arrived, followed by an ambulance. Everything was a blur after that, while various medical professionals worked on my father. Eventually they stretchered him downstairs and into the ambulance. The paramedic told Mum that he was fighting for his life, and needed to get to hospital as soon as was humanly possible. And off they sped into the distance, sirens blazing.

Mum followed, but asked me to stay at home and ring Julie. Luckily some friends came round, and helped me to stay calm while I was waiting for news. Julie phoned after about an hour, to say that she'd got my message and was on her way to Bournemouth Hospital. She had quite a journey ahead of her.

I cancelled all my business appointments for the rest of the day, and settled down to wait for news of my father. Eventually Mum phoned, and said that he was stable, although he would have to stay in hospital for at least a week, to recuperate and to have various tests.

After the results came through, Dad was told that he needed to go to Guy's Hospital in London for an operation, and he was admitted for a quadruple bypass in October. It was another very tense day. I went out to Mudeford, to watch the boats and listen to my radio.

I kept thinking back to all the happy times I'd had with my family in the past. I tortured myself with the thought that the stress caused by my illness had given Dad his heart problem. I knew that feeling guilty wouldn't help though, so I tried to relax while I waited – and thank goodness it was good news again. Dad got through his bypass, and came home soon afterwards, with a video of the operation for us all to watch (if we wanted to!). He had to rest afterwards, sitting in an armchair in front of the television. His friend often came over to watch TV with him – usually Manchester United games, which kept them both happy.

I was soon distracted by a new Motability car – the Rover 25. I loved this car – it is still my favourite out of all those that I have owned. It was sporty and yet economical, and it it looked good inside and out. It really was a superb car.

I didn't celebrate my birthday in October – apart from anything else, Dad didn't need any extra excitement in his life, as he was still convalescing. He steadily improved though, and on Christmas Day he treated us to his usual speech. 'Merry Christmas to Jim the Tin Man!'

I toasted him, and we all raised our glasses, knowing how lucky we were that he still held his place in the centre of our little family.

I was very busy at the start of 2005, building castles and making signs. One morning I set off to see Paddy, my signwriter, at his Bournemouth studio. I was in my car, driving along the dual carriageway, when I completely lost my concentration and became confused and disorientated.

Luckily I retained enough sense to immediately pull my car over onto the hard shoulder and stop. A police car that happened to be nearby pulled alongside, and one of the policemen got out. He asked what was wrong, and I told him that I had lost my memory. He looked very concerned.

I knew that something was very wrong – I could see bright white lights ahead of me and could not understand why. I felt extremely light-headed and I didn't have any idea where I had been driving to. However, when the policeman asked my name and address I knew that immediately, which was a relief for us both!

A paramedic was called to the scene. He checked my blood pressure and heart and found nothing wrong. Then I realised I felt better – I had rallied round. It was most peculiar. The paramedic and the policemen all said that I should go straight to my GP, so after going home and telling Mum what had happened I rang the surgery. The GP must have realised that something serious was afoot, because he told me to come right over.

The GP could also find nothing immediately wrong, but

he sent me for blood tests at Christchurch Hospital. Three days later, the surgery rang, asking me to go in urgently to discuss my blood test results. Mum came with me to the surgery for support.

'Is it cancer, doctor?' I blurted out as soon as I got into the consulting room.

'No,' he said, 'It's not that bad. But you do have a serious case of anaemia. Your levels of Vitamin B12 are incredibly low, and we need to act fast'.

The doctor explained the treatment for my condition – he said that I would need to have six injections of Vitamin B12 over the next fortnight. That would help me, but it would take a full three months for me to get back to normal. He said that I should drink Guinness and eat Marmite to speed up the process!

The doctor then asked if I was a vegetarian. I told him that yes, I had been a vegetarian for more than twenty years without any noticeable ill-effects. I had given up meat because I found it difficult to digest, and it was giving me stomach cramps. I had not really missed it in my diet, I told him.

The doctor then told me that the stomach cramps were probably partly to do with my Morquio's condition. He said that it was sensible of me to have given up meat, but that to be a healthy vegetarian you have to watch your diet carefully and take vitamin supplements. He could have simply given me medication to help me digest the meat more effectively, he said, if only I had asked!

I was very weak for the next three months, just as the

doctor had forecast. I was very tired and also dizzy and confused at times. I suffered from stomach cramps and disturbed vision, and a strange feeling like pinpricks on my scalp which I thought of as 'a rainstorm'. I learned that this sensation was due to a lack of oxygen to the blood cells in the brain.

It was the summer now, so I was able to rest in the garden. I lay in my deckchair listening to the radio. My sign writer looked after the business for me, and after the three months period of convalescence was up I was relieved to find that I felt much brighter again. I had a blood test to check my progress, and the doctor told me formally that I could start working again. He said, however, that I would need to have an injection of vitamin B12 every three months for life. If not, he told me, it would be curtains for me!

I hate these injections, but I have no choice but to submit to them. I was shocked to learn that this situation arose because of vegetarianism, something that I thought would make me stronger and healthier. I am hoping that this book will help to spread the message to anyone who is a vegetarian or thinking of becoming one, to get advice from a doctor or nutritionist.

Chapter Twenty-Eight
Fire!

My sister Julie called one day to see how I was. I told her that I was recovering nicely. 'What's that racket in the background?' I asked.

'It's the British Grand Prix,' she told me.

'I didn't know you liked Formula One!' I exclaimed. 'How strange'.

'Oh yes,' she said, 'I've been watching it for years. I love the speed of the cars. Don't forget you support Brazil – that may sound strange to some people'.

'Well, you'd better drive off now, before the other drivers overtake you!' I said, and we laughed. I miss my sister sometimes – it is a pity she doesn't live closer, but it is always good to speak to her on the phone.

In October that year it was the first anniversary of Dad's heart operation. Mum encouraged him to socialise, and this helped, but he was still not quite as hale and hearty as he used to be. Every day made a difference though, and I was so proud of him for managing to regain his health.

On my birthday, I decided to go fishing at Clay Pool on the River Stour. I was going to cycle, but found that my back and ribs were too stiff to allow me to mount my bike. I was really upset, and started swearing at the bike, then pushed it to the ground and walked off into the house angrily. By the time Mum came to see what was the matter, I was in tears.

'Don't give up, son,' she said. 'Try again'.

I took strength from her words, and I did manage to get up onto the bike eventually. I slowly rode around the block – but it was painful, not just in my joints, but with my hands straining to hold the handlebars. When I finally arrived home I stopped at the side gate, and found that I could not dismount the bike. There was nobody at home to help, and I began to panic. Eventually I slid off onto a tall flower pot. It was a great relief – I'd thought I was going to be stuck on that bike all day. So that was a memorable birthday, but for all the wrong reasons!

In November, I was referred to the Royal Bournemouth Hospital to see the orthopaedic specialist. This was much easier to get to than Southampton General Hospital, and the car parking system was far better too. The appointment went well, and I was told that my treatment could be fully transferred to Bournemouth. My surgical shoes play an important part in my life – without them I would be pretty much immobile, so anything which improves their provision is very welcome to me.

I painted another Christmas display this year – Mickey Mouse and Minnie Mouse out carol singing with Donald Duck. Christmas Day was just the same as ever. I was very fond of our traditions - Mum's marvellous cooking, Dad's famous speech, and my Christmas pictures.

In January 2006, I finally accepted that my bicycle had to go. My disabilities were worsening and I knew that I would never be able to ride it again. I had named my bike, which was specially designed for me, Olympian. I am not ashamed to say that I actually kissed it goodbye and thanked it for giving me strength and freedom, before it went on its last journey, to the tip.

In June, Germany hosted the World Cup, which was always a big event on my calendar. I was watching Brazil, hoping that they would win their sixth title. They got through to the quarter-finals, but then lost to France, which was a disappointment, but as I will always maintain, Brazil are still the best!

In August, disaster struck. The weather was very warm, and I spent a lot of time working outdoors. Early one morning, I heard crackling coming from the garage of the house next door. It became quite loud, and eventually I went inside to ask Mum what she thought it might be.

Our neighbour was due to move house, and Mum said she thought the noise was probably her packing up her belongings. So I carried on working, paying no attention to the crackling sound, which eventually stopped. I went out to a party that night and had a great time, arriving home just after midnight. I parked my car on the driveway, and was surprised to hear that the crackling noise had started again. 'Surely she can't still be packing, at this time of night,' I thought.

I was tired though, so did not try to investigate, but headed straight to my bedroom. I opened the windows wide, because the night air was warm, and as I got into bed I was already drifting off to sleep. Suddenly, there was a huge explosion. I thought at first that it was thunder, but then Mum came storming into my room, shouting, 'Anton, fire! Fire! Get out of the house, quickly!'

I was still trying to get dressed, while Dad had made his way outside to see what was happening. When he saw that our neighbour's house and garage were ablaze, he called the fire brigade. He banged on the front door of the neighbour's house to wake her, but she was nowhere to be seen. The guttering on our house was alight by now and was spreading across to my bedroom windows. I just managed to get my clothes on as more explosions occurred, and I headed down the stairs like a flash!

Mum had been waiting for me by our front door, which is at the side of our house. She and I could not get out to the street in front, because of the explosions, which were caused by the asbestos roof of our neighbour's garage. Small pieces of blazing asbestos were shooting around like popcorn. So we went in the other direction, to the bottom of our garden, and took shelter behind Dad's shed. The asbestos fireballs were spraying into our garden and that of the other neighbours – it was quite frightening.

Mum was still dressed in her nightclothes, and was shaking with fear, and coughing from having inhaled smoke. I took my T-shirt off and soaked it in the garden water tank, then gave it to my Mum to hold over her nose and mouth. Meanwhile, Dad was using a garden hose to stop the fire from spreading to our roof.

The fire was spreading, to our caravan and the neighbour's bedroom roof. The heat and smoke from the fire were overpowering now, and I was worried that Mum and I would suffocate, down behind the garden shed. I had started to plan our escape, thinking that I would use my built-up shoe to smash our way through the fence into the neighbour's garden – but then thankfully the Christchurch Fire Brigade arrived.

Once the fire was under control, a fire officer checked that it was safe for us to return home. He spoke to us about what might have caused the fire, and when I told him about the crackling noises I had heard earlier in the day, he realised that it was due to the fridge freezer which was kept in our neighbour's garage.

We wondered why our smoke alarms hadn't worked, and were puzzled when he said that it was because the fire had produced a 'different kind of smoke'. Surely smoke was smoke, and the alarms were supposed to detect it? Later, another fire officer admitted that they really did not know why our alarms had not worked – he was very sympathetic and helped us fill in a report for the household insurance company.

When Mum and I headed out through our garden into the street we were greeted by a street full of neighbours who had been concerned for our safety. It was very moving. Although we were not hurt there had been a lot of damage to the house and the summerhouse, and to our caravan. My sister Julie always made me promise to ring her in any emergency, so I phoned to tell her what had happened. She travelled down immediately, arriving that night while the firemen were still working, which was very sweet of her.

The next morning our street was full of men in white protective overalls, gathering the scattered asbestos. The fire officer re-visited too, which was thoughtful. However, because the fire was declared to be accidental, Mum and Dad were not due any compensation from the neighbour, so they had to pay the excess on their own insurance policy before they could have any work done on the house.

Two months later the bulk of the damage was fixed – the neighbour's garage and a section of her house was rebuilt, and we had replacement double glazed windows, new guttering and so on. Mum and Dad's car was also slightly damaged, as was mine. I called the Motability service to tell them what had happened, and they were very kind, wanting to ensure that I had not been harmed in any way.

The year was winding down now. I was forty-eight in October – sometimes I wonder where all the years have gone! In November I started work on my Christmas display – Winnie the Pooh and friends. And on Christmas Day, with just the three of us for dinner, Dad made a short speech thanking the Fire Brigade for saving our lives.

I had a lot of Christmas gifts and cards from people I had never met, who had seen my castles or Christmas displays, or heard of me through my charity work, and I found this heart-warming. I did my best to put the house fire out of my mind, although the incident left me with a serious fear of fire. Even now I can't bear to be near a bonfire, a log fire, or even a barbecue or lighted candle.

Mum came into my garage studio early in 2007, and was concerned to find me in tears. 'What's the matter?' she asked. 'Are you in pain?'

'No,' I said, 'But I do need to talk to you about something'.

We went inside together, and Mum made me a cup of tea. Then I told her that I was bored, lonely and depressed. I did not know how these feelings had crept up on me – I had been happy working hard, making castles and signs, but suddenly I was feeling very isolated.

'I thought this might happen,' Mum told me. 'Your Dad and I have noticed that you have been working a lot and not socialising much recently. It is important to keep a balance of work and play in your life. How about joining a club of some sort, to make some new friends?'

I decided to take a day off work and go for a drive, as I often did when I needed to think a problem over. I ended up by the water in Southampton, watching the container ships come in to dock from the Solent. I put the radio on, tuned into a French radio station and ate some currant buns. I felt better already!

Then I heard somebody singing, 'Happy talking, talking, happy talk!' I looked out of my window and was amazed to see my old friend Declan, or 'Captain Sensible' as I used to style him. 'Hello Anton,' he said merrily. 'Are you here on business?'

'Sort of,' I smiled. 'How are you?'

'Fantastic!' he replied. 'That project you helped me with is going to be built by the end of this year. I never did thank you properly for all the time you spent with me working on it. Oh, and this will make you laugh. Remember how you drove around on my lawn mower taking photos?'

'How could I forget?' I said.

'Well, after you left, I tried to put the mower away, but the steering wheel jammed. I landed head first in the river. The tide was out luckily, but I got plastered in mud'.

When I finally stopped laughing, Declan asked me out for lunch. We had a meal at the Solent Cafe. As we were due to leave, he said, 'I hope all those people don't scratch my car'. There was a group clustered around his vehicle and I soon saw why.

'Good grief!' I exclaimed. 'You've got a white Lotus Spirit, just like the one James Bond drove in The Spy Who Loved Me. You lucky so-and-so!'

He walked with me to my car, and we said goodbye. Declan thanked me again for helping him – but it was only after he'd gone that I saw he had left an envelope in my car, with a large cheque in it. He was a very generous man.

I stayed on in the car park after my friend drove off in his Lotus. I was still thinking hard about my future, and then finally I had an idea. I reached home late that afternoon, and Mum asked me whether I had come to any decisions about how to improve my life.

'I have a great idea,' I told her. 'I am going to apply to join the fundraising team of The Children's Trust'.

'But it's over a hundred miles away!' she objected.

I was not to be deterred, and immediately fired off a letter to the Trust. I received a reply just a few days later – my application had been accepted! I would be a local volunteer fundraiser, working with a lady who managed fundraising throughout Hampshire, Wiltshire and Dorset.

A few days later I received a call from my manager. She had a beautiful speaking voice. 'This is SJ from The Children's Trust,' she told me, 'I would like to arrange to come and meet you, please'.

We agreed to meet at my house, and I told Mum that we would probably need to roll out the red carpet as our visitor spoke like royalty. She turned out to be a delightful person, and she put me at my ease immediately. We talked about the Trust, which caters for children with multiple disabilities and brain injuries, and we chatted about my time at Tadworth Court.

SJ told me that she needed to raise a large amount of money each year, and that we would have to work hard to reach our target, and I said that I was ready to do whatever it took. I was really excited to be involved with The Children's Trust. I showed SJ my castles, and she was really impressed. I suggested that I could display a castle at a local supermarket, with a bucket collection, and she agreed.

Before SJ left she gave me two collection boxes and lots of leaflets about the Trust, so that I could start fundraising immediately. 'Don't worry, I won't let you down,' I told her. I took a box down to a local newsagents, who agreed to keep it on the counter. I still keep a collection box there today, and every month I collect and bank the takings. That first month I raised £7, which may not seem like a lot of money, but I felt was a good start. It all adds up, over the years.

In March I began to build a new castle for The Children's Trust. I fixed it on wheels to make it portable. It took me the rest of the year to complete –

you don't want to know how many cardboard tubes, cereal boxes and shoe boxes, and how much masking tape, papier mache and PVA glue I used. Blue Peter have got nothing on me!

Of course, building the castle took so long because I also had to continue my paid work, signwriting. I finished it eventually though, and it was a work of art, if I say so myself – a replica of a medieval castle, painted red, blue and black.

I did have a small birthday celebration that year, which was thoroughly enjoyable. Next year I would be fifty, and it was amazing to think that I had reached such an age – far in advance of what my parents had once been told would be possible.

That year I was far too busy working on my castle to paint a Christmas display. I was looking forward to embarking on my bucket collection events. Christmas Day was a marvellous care-free event. I reflected back on my life – I was almost fifty and still living at home, but as happy as I had ever been in my life. I realised that I was a very fortunate person to be so secure in my family and home.

Chapter Twenty-Nine
Building Castles

Early in 2008 I finally finished making The Children's Trust Fundraising Castle. I decided to display it on our driveway. I carefully raised the garage door as high as it would go, and pushed the castle out – but, to my dismay, as I did so one of the large towers with all its spires, completely snapped off. I had built the castle eight inches too tall to fit through!

I was really cross with myself, but I rallied, wheeled it back into the garage, and pondered my next move. Eventually I picked up my sketch book and drove down to Mudeford Quay to have a good think. My mobile phone rang just as I got to the Quay. It was a lady, who introduced herself as Hilary. 'I have heard that you are a local craftsman, and I was wondering whether you could make my daughter a crown for her school play?' she asked. 'She will need it in time for Easter'.

'I'm sure I can do that,' I told her. 'Come and see me tomorrow, and we'll discuss it properly'.

As I switched my phone off, I was still thinking about the crown, and about my broken castle, and suddenly I had a brainwave. I could make a small crown to fix to the top of the tower! That would tidy up the castle and avoid having to start on my project all over again! By the time Hilary turned up the next morning to talk about her daughter's crown, I had already fixed my castle, and I was delighted. I told her that I would make the crown free of charge, as she had helped me out with a major problem.

In February, I travelled to Tadworth to meet up with SJ

and be introduced to the rest of The Children's Trust Fundraising Team. I was shown around the grounds of Tadworth Court, which were as magical as ever and seemed largely unchanged. Various new buildings were dotted about, which had been built to cater for the needs of the disabled children. The staff seemed as friendly and helpful as ever, and I felt very much at home there.

The Children's Trust was established to provide care, education and therapy for children with a variety of disabilities and other health conditions. I saw some of these children, seriously ill and struggling to cope with the difficulties they faced, and this made me feel sad. I felt that they were in the best hands possible at Tadworth Court though.

I had a busy day, and quickly understood how vital the work of the Fundraising Department was. There were so many projects lined up for the staff at Tadworth – but all of it was dependent on the efforts of these fundraisers. And part of the responsibility was now mine! The time flew by, and soon my friend arrived to collect me. I was sad to leave, but felt that I'd had a really enjoyable and worthwhile day out.

Our local police constable, Martin Sparks, is a friend of our family. He is a Police Community Support Officer (PCSO) and his duty is to tackle anti-social behaviour and other issues affecting quality of life in the locality. One day Martin told me that he planned to run a half marathon, and asked if he could help to raise funds for The Children's Trust. I told SJ, who was very pleased. Martin and I both worked to get plenty of sponsors and he was very well supported by family, friends, and his colleagues at Christchurch Police Station.

On the day of the run, my parents and I watched from Bournemouth cliff top. 'What on earth is Martin wearing?' I asked. 'He looks like mobile wallpaper, with those red and white stripes'.

'He's a Southampton football supporter,' my Mum told me. 'And don't you dare take the mickey out of him for it!'

Martin finished in good time that day, and he raised more than £350 for the Trust. I was really grateful to him for his efforts.

In June the new fundraising castle went on tour, to the David English Sports Centre. Hundreds of children took part in a fun run, and enjoyed the stalls and rides. It was a windy day, but very sunny. SJ, who met Mum and I there, had set up a gazebo. We had a good time, working together on a bucket collection for the castle, and we stayed out all day.

In September the New Forest District Council gave me a day licence for a bucket collection at the nearby Ringwood Shopping Centre. I set up my pitch at 8am outside Sainsbury's, and the manager of the supermarket was very kind and helpful after I showed him my ID from The Children's Trust.

Mum and I sat on a wall, holding our buckets. Surprisingly, it was against the law for us to shake them. Many people gave us change, and many others hurried past on their way. My most surprising 'customer' was a tramp who turned up pushing a bicycle with bags tied all over the handlebars. He dug his hand into his pocket and pulled out some coins which he put into the bucket. I thanked him for his trouble and he smiled, gave me a 'thumbs up' sign, and pushed his bicycle off again. I was really touched by the fact that somebody with so little had the kindness to give to others.

It was a busy morning – first a photographer from the Bournemouth Daily Echo turned up to take my picture, and next a reporter from that paper called my mobile, to ask about the castle. 'How much are you hoping to raise today?' he asked, and I told him that £100 would be great.

By the end of the day, the collection bucket was so heavy that I could hardly get it into the car, and when we reached home I had to ask Dad to lift it onto the kitchen table for me. I was sure that we had raised a fortune!

To my disappointment though, the bucket contained mostly copper coins, so although it looked and felt like a lot of money it only added up to about £45. As SJ said though, when I phoned the next day to give her the bad news, 'Every penny counts!' She said that Mum and I had done a great job and thanked us both profusely.

On the 17th October it was my fiftieth birthday – at last! For my present, Mum and Dad had thought up something original – they adopted a tiger in my name from the World Wildlife Fund! We had an open house at home all day, and many friends came by to visit.

On Sunday the 20th, we had a lunch party at the Royal Exeter Hotel for my special friends and family. I received lots of cards and some lovely presents, including albums by Demis Roussos, Kate Ryan and Sandrine Francois. My dear friend Ric bought me a book on famous castles – he had inscribed, 'Keep Going!' inside the front cover.

The year soon came to a close. I remember that the start of 2009 was freezing. Very low temperatures and heavy snowfall caused disruption across the UK, and many of our local schools were closed. I felt privileged that I was able to continue to work out in my garage studio, with central heating to keep me warm.

That spring I was really pleased when Martin Sparks told me that he wanted to raise money for The Children's Trust again, this time by running the London Marathon. He told me that he planned to dress as Banana Man, which I found very funny. On 26th April, the day of the Marathon, Mum Dad and I were glued to the TV screen. We tried hard to see Martin – but were flummoxed by the fact that there were many other charity fun runners also dressed as Banana Man!

The Children's Trust were one of the Marathon's official charities that year, which meant that their team included more than 650 runners. I spotted many runners wearing The Children's Trust T-shirt. I really wanted to see my friend Geoffrey, who was running as Tadworth the Hound, The Children's Trust Mascot – unfortunately though, it was just too crowded to spot him.

Martin called me when the run was over. He had managed to complete the course in good time, and raised a grand total of £859, moving the Trust well in the direction of their £1 million target. Martin struggled to walk for several days afterwards, as his feet had broken out in painful blisters, but he managed to make it round to my house to show me his Marathon Medal. I was really proud.

The Children's Trust celebrated their 25th Anniversary,

with a number of special events. A new residential rehabilitation centre and hydrotherapy pool was opened at Tadworth, and I was glad to think that I had contributed, in my small way, to this great achievement.

Spurred on, I came up with another fundraising idea – Charity Hoopla Castles. The castles came with a set of rings and a display board, and proved to be a great way to raise money. I still use them at fundraising events now, and rent them out for use to other charities too.

Other castles I'd built were sent to France and Germany for Arts and Crafts exhibitions and window displays. I was in full production at that time. I liked working outside on my driveway – I have a long-standing habit of waving to helicopters as they fly past. One day I had a close shave – the Red Arrows aero display team flew past while I was working outside on my driveway. I was so shocked by the noise, and by how low they flew, that I literally fell off my chair, and was covered in blue paint!

I went inside to tell Mum what had happened. I was very indignant, but she made me laugh, saying that I was lucky to have enjoyed a free personal air display. 'And at least you're not hurt,' she reminded me. Only my dignity was wounded!

In 2010 I received bad news - Paddy, my subcontracted sign-writer, had to retire for health reasons. My health was suffering too – my disability was worsening, and arthritis had set in firmly and was affecting all my bone joints. The pain was so bad that at times I could hardly even hold a paint brush. There were days when I could not even walk to my car, much less attempt to drive it. Every day was a struggle but I refused to give up.

I was worried about how my business would survive without poor Paddy, but help arrived in the form of Ross. Ross had his own signwriting business, but was willing to help me to keep mine going. We had a lot in common, and we soon became firm friends. Ross helped me to build a new website for my business, Purewell Signwriters and Anton's Eurocastles. He did a good job – it was very colourful, with a home page about how I started my business, and with plenty of pictures.

In March that year I decided to design and build fourteen small fantasy castles and one very tall slimline castle, with castors. I used the Echo, our local paper, and PVA glue to make papier mache and was very pleased with the result. The thin newspaper soaked up the PVA fast, and then I worked it into a sticky paste with my fingers. I found that I could make very effective designs in this way.

In April the TV newsreader announced that a cloud of volcanic ash in Iceland had caused the closure of the airspace over the UK and Northern and Western Europe. I was dismayed, because this meant that I could not work on my castles outside – when I tried I got coughing fits and had to head back into my garage studio and shut the door.

The volcano ash blurred our blue skies to a light brown colour, which was quite alarming. Fortunately it all cleared soon enough and the UK was back to normal service.

In May 2010 there was another general election, which had a very unusual outcome. No party won an absolute majority of seats, so the Conservatives and Liberal Democrats combined forces, and Britain had a coalition government for the first time since Winston Churchill's wartime government.

There was also another World Cup this year – but I was disappointed that Brazil only made it to the quarter-finals. Spain became the world champions for the first time, beating the Netherlands in the final by one goal to nil.

I was not totally disappointed though and I kept my Brazilian flag flying for some time after the competition was over. I was pleased because it had been announced that Brazil were due to host the next FIFA cup in 2014. That was something to look forward to!

At the beginning of August I started to suffer from terrible pain in my left hip. The arthritis was getting a grip, now that I could not cycle to grind it off. Things rapidly worsened – I started to get muscle spasms in my left leg, travelling right up to my buttocks.

I went to see my GP, who sent me for immediate X-rays at Christchurch Hospital. The results confirmed that my hip joints were solid with arthritis, which had caused the muscle spasms in my leg. He gave me a prescription to ease the spasms, and also recommended Glucosamine with Chondroitin to reduce the joint pains and stiffness. The GP also referred me to the specialist at the Royal Bournemouth Hospital, but warned that there was a two month waiting list.

Meanwhile, I attended the Studland Country Fair, taking my hoopla castle along to raise money for The Children's Trust. The weather was sunny and warm and we were bombarded by wasps in the field where we had set up our gazebo. It was a good day though – there was lots to see at the fair, including food stalls, arts and crafts and a fantastic dog show. Mum, Dad and Dad's friend Rodney all helped out, and we had an enjoyable time and raised £80 for the Trust from the Hoopla castle. I also displayed my small castles in the gazebo and sold one of them (I donated this money to the Trust too).

In September I got a new Motability car, a light blue Ford Focus. I was very pleased with it. My birthday was not very exciting this year though, since I was in too much discomfort to enjoy myself very much. In fact, I was finding it increasingly difficult to walk.

The appointment to see the orthopaedic consultant in Bournemouth finally came through in November. He explained that the worsening arthritis now meant that I had very little movement left in my hip joints, and that although he could operate, this might not improve matters and could even worsen them.

I immediately replied that I would rather not undergo the operation. I couldn't face the thought of things going wrong, especially because of the worry this would cause to my parents. The consultant understood, but told me to make sure that my surgical shoes were always correctly balanced, and said I should contact him immediately if I had any more problems.

The consultant also told me that I should lose weight, as a matter of urgency, to reduce the pressure on my hips. He also said that I should keep taking the Glucosamine, and after a few weeks I did feel that things were improving and that I had increased mobility in my hips.

Christmas was approaching fast, and I managed to complete my Christmas display – it was a pantomime picture, themed around Pinnochio. However, I then suffered severe back pain, and the doctor said to my surprise that this was caused by constipation, which had been set off by the other medication I had been prescribed for the muscle spasms. The doctor gave me some more pills to counteract it, but I was not at all well or happy. Even on Christmas day I was feeling rotten, and was not in the mood to eat my meal. However, Mum's Christmas pudding soon sorted things out (enough said!)

The start of the following year was a bit slack work-wise, so I decided to start writing notes about my life, hoping to put it all together into an autobiography one day. I went to see one of my old school friends, who now ran a Bed and Breakfast business, Castle Lodge in Highcliffe, and she allocated me a table in her lounge at which I could sit and write. I was pleased with the arrangement and soon settled into my new routine, writing at Castle Lodge each morning during the week.

In April I visited The Children's Trust at Tadworth Court again, to meet SJ and Karen, who also works for the Trust. I decided to travel in style this time, and hired myself a chauffeur driven Mercedes! It was a good decision – the driver was very friendly and helpful, and good company too, and the journey passed quickly.

At Tadworth, Karen pushed me around in a wheelchair. I saw the old ZMA and ZMB wards, which brought back some memories. The buildings had been modified and were really well kept – they still had some of the original features, such as the patio. Karen took me to a new building too, where the children received music therapy. There was a grand piano there, and Karen said I could play it, so I did a rendition of Greensleeves.

The Children's Trust was thriving, and I was glad that I had become involved with them. Clearly a lot of children were benefiting from the work of this marvellous charity. It was a warm sunny day, the atmosphere at Tadworth Court was as magical as ever and I felt really happy as I was shown around, although as always I was sad to leave.

I had several health problems at that time, including difficulties with mobility. The GP sent me for blood tests, which came back clear. He then advised me to contact Social Services, and when they arrived at my home several weeks later, they saw that I needed serious help. I couldn't use the bath or shower, I had problems getting in and out of my bed and armchair, and even struggled to get over the front doorstep. They said they would see what they could do to help, and I settled down to await developments.

On the 29th April it was a big day for the country – Prince William married Catherine Middleton at Westminster Abbey in London. It was a beautiful wedding, and I enjoyed watching it on the television. There were street parties all over the country, and I was really sorry that I did not feel well enough to join in.

In May I visited my GP yet again, to complain about the residual catarrh in my nose and throat, which I was finding very upsetting. He made me an appointment at the hospital to investigate this, and he also referred me for an Echocardiogram (an ultrasound of the heart). However, he told me that there was a long waiting list for these procedures.

Meanwhile, I could no longer work outside, as even the pollen from flowers had started to affect my throat. I could not use glue to build my castles either, because it worsened my condition. I stayed indoors throughout the summer, trying to keep my symptoms at bay with the help of a nasal spray, but it was really not an easy time. Luckily I could still build hoopla castles, and Anton's Euro Castles operated as usual. My friend agreed to run my sign writing business until I felt well enough to take over again.

In May, the Social Services suggested I should have a care support line. I pay a fixed annual fee for this and it gives us all peace of mind. Then in June a stair lift was installed, which seemed like a godsend – until it went wrong! The stair lift started to make a banging noise, then vibrating wildly, nearly throwing me off in transit and causing great pain that lasted for days. Attempts were made to mend the thing, but one day it stopped working entirely – half way up the stairs with me on board!

Time after time, attempts were made to fix that stair lift. The last straw came one night when the three of us waited all day for a technician who finally arrived just a quarter of an hour before midnight. We were all shattered, but we hadn't dared to cancel the appointment and go to bed, in case we were never given another appointment.

So that was that – we told the firm to take the contraption away as it was not fit for purpose, and I was back to struggling up and down the stairs with the help of my parents. They now couldn't leave the house for more than an hour or two at a time because I was pretty much immobilised.

I struggled on and in July I used my care allowance to buy myself a new wheelchair, from All Mobility Care in Christchurch. In August Social Services arranged for the installation of a new electronic toilet, which doubled as a bidet, and undoubtedly made my life easier. This was fitted by a very good company, Gerberit Aqua Clean Care.

I was still fundraising, and in September I organised a quiz night for The Children's Trust, at Boscombe Cliff Bowling Club. It went very well, and hot on its heels I organised a live band, Uptown Traffic, to play at the Highcliffe Social and Sports Club. That was a great evening out, and a great fundraiser too.

Because of all the problems with my first stair lift, in October Social Services authorised us to seek the guidance of Stannah, the best known firm in the business. I was invited to visit their showroom in Andover, and treated like royalty there. We ordered a stair lift, and were told that it would be installed as soon as possible.

I celebrated my birthday quietly again that year. In November I had the Echocardiogram to check my heart function, which was fine - although I was told again that I really should lose weight to ease the burden on my body. That is always easier said than done though!

Later that month I had another appointment at the Royal Bournemouth, for my nose and throat problem. After I was given a local anaesthetic to numb the area, a tiny camera was inserted through my nose and threaded down into my throat. I could have nothing to eat or drink for five hours and I talked like Donald Duck for a long time afterwards – it was a really unpleasant experience. To my relief though, nothing untoward was found.

Two days later, at the end of November, I had a CT scan done at the same hospital. This felt strange and intimidating, like being asked to put my head inside a washing machine, but fortunately it was over in a couple of minutes. I was getting fed up now of being poked and prodded, but knew that I was lucky to get my health thoroughly checked in this way. I was told that the results of the CT scan would not be known until the next year.

In December, Stannah installed my new stair lift and this time everything went smoothly. We have received a very efficient and professional service from Stannah, who have a depot just a mile from our house – it really could not be better. Also in December, a wet room was installed in our house, to make it easier for me to wash. It took less than two weeks from start to finish, and was an example of really brilliant workmanship by the company who fitted it, Mears. The only hitch was that in order to use the shower I needed special waterproof shoes to keep me balanced, because my right leg is a lot shorter than the left. My GP wrote to the Prosthetics and Orthotics Centre at Bournemouth Hospital, but yet again I was told that I would have to wait a while before I heard from them.

Meanwhile I came up with a solution for myself – I showered while wearing one of my old pairs of leather shoes. I knew that my surgical shoe maker would not be very pleased if he found out, but I was quite confident that nobody was going to tell him!

After our Christmas dinner that year, Dad made his usual speech, thanking the Social Services, the GP and hospitals, and all the companies who had made my life easier. Everything finally seemed to be ticking along again after a rocky year.

To round the year off, Mum, Dad and I watched the French New Year's Eve party, Bonne Grande on La Monde's TV5 Europe. This is always a really good show, hosted by Patrick Sebastian and incorporating cabaret, magicians, illusionists and so on. When that show finished, we watched the English New Year fireworks display over Big Ben. And then on New Year's Day itself, we turned BBC2 on, and watched and listened to the Vienna Philharmonic Orchestra performing their annual celebratory concert of waltzes, polkas and marches. What a cultured lot we are – and thank goodness for the television, which enables us to be so!

Chapter Thirty
A Reunion

2012 started badly. My GP called to tell me that he'd received a letter from the Prosthetics Centre at Bournemouth Hospital, saying that they could not provide me with waterproof shoes for use in my shower. They said that no such product existed and that it would be too difficult to make. They cited health and safety reasons in their letter, assuring the GP that cost was not the influencing factor in their decision. So I was stuck – no waterproof shoes and no prospect of any. Meanwhile, having no other choice, I continued to shower in my old leather shoes.

One day I was chatting to Rosie Groves, the wife of my old friend Garry. She asked how my book was coming on, and I told her that although I had made many pages of notes I was struggling to write it. 'Really, I could do with a ghost writer,' I told her. 'But I have no idea how to go about finding such a person'.

Not long afterwards I received a call from a woman called Louise, who said that she had been given my number by Rosie. 'I hear you are looking for a ghost writer,' she said. 'I might be able to help'.

Louise and I arranged to meet in March, at a clothes show that I had organised to raise money for The Children's Trust. Fittingly, the show was due to be held at Castle Lodge, where I had been working steadily on my book over the previous year. I put down the phone feeling a lot happier, knowing that at last I might have found someone who could help me with my writing.

Meanwhile, I had a call from Rosemarie Glithero.

Rosemarie works for The Children's Trust at Tadworth Court as a Leisure and Activities Co-ordinator. She arranges outings for the children, as well as activities and events on-site. She takes the children to theme parks, theatres and even wheelchair ice-skating and often drives the minibus herself on these occasions. She is one remarkably caring action lady!

I had met Rosemarie through my fund-raising work for the Trust. We had talked about the time I had spent at Tadworth Court in 1973, and she had called now to tell me that she had found a nurse who had looked after me in those days. Rosemarie said she would pass my number on, and just after nine o'clock that evening the phone rang. 'Hello,' I said tentatively.

'Hi Anton. My name is Maggie Tamplin,' said the voice on the other end of the line. 'I used to be a nurse on ZMB ward in 1973. You were there then – I wonder if you remember me?'

'I certainly do,' I said. 'I recognised your voice straight away. I can't believe that I am talking to you, after all these years'.

Maggie had worked at Tadworth Court when it still belonged to Great Ormond Street Hospital. She had left to bring up her family, and then returned when Tadworth was taken over by The Children's Trust. In all my visits I had never realised that Maggie still worked there!

It was really good to talk to her – and the next thing I heard was that Rob Wood, Marketing and Communications Manager of The Children's Trust, had arranged for Maggie and I to meet up at Tadworth Court in mid-February. It would be our first meeting for more than forty years – we would have our picture taken together, and I was to expect a call from the Trust Press Office the next day.

On the appointed day, February 13th, a friend drove me to Tadworth Court, to meet Maggie Tamplin and Rosemarie Glithero. It was a cold day and when we arrived, the ground was covered in a deep layer of snow. My friend started to get my wheelchair out of the car – but meanwhile Maggie drove up. She stopped her car, then caught sight of me and rushed over to give me a big hug, leaving the engine still running in all her excitement!

Rosemarie, Maggie, my friend and I then headed to the restaurant inside Tadworth Court, for a cup of tea and a chat. Maggie had brought her photo album, and she showed me a picture of two little boys, who I recognised as Mark and Sinclair.

Then Rob Wood arrived to take the pictures, for which Maggie and I posed outside. Rosemarie and Maggie then took us to see ZMA and ZMB. I told my friend all about the time I had spent at Tadworth Court and she was fascinated. Maggie showed us the old operating room, which was now a kitchen, and the plaster room, now used for storage. The memories all came flooding back.

A lot of improvements had been made since my time, and all the buildings now had wonderful modern facilities for the disabled children. Rosemarie and Maggie took us to see the new swimming pool, which was truly fantastic, and the tree house which had been designed to be accessed by children in wheelchairs. Apparently Mr Tumble from the BBC CBeebies programme had filmed here, and of course the children had loved him.

'I love Mr Tumble too,' I admitted, and Rosemarie smiled and said that she was also a fan.

Maggie then showed us Mulberry House, where she worked. This accommodation unit gives respite care. Some children with severe disabilities and complex health needs require round the clock care, which can be exhausting for their families. Respite care gives the parents a short break to recharge their batteries, knowing that their children can enjoy their time away too, in a safe setting with others of their age. It is a blessing for everyone concerned.

The four of us had lunch together in the restaurant and Maggie and I agreed to keep in contact. I told her and Rosemarie that I was working on my autobiography, which was about my life, especially my disability and the challenges I had faced and overcome. They were so pleased to hear that all the proceeds from the book would be going to The Children's Trust and to Great Ormond Street Hospital.

It had always been difficult to leave Tadworth Court, and this time was no exception. I said my farewells sadly, and set off with my friend. The next day a lady from The Children's Trust Press Office called and asked all about my meeting with Maggie, and suddenly the story seemed to be everywhere – in the local newspaper, The Children's Trust Website, even on Facebook! 'Anton meets up with Nurse after 40 Years' the headlines declared. It was all very exciting.

In March, Louise (the ghostwriter) and I met at Castle

382

Lodge, at the Second Hand Rose designer Clothes Sale that I had organised in aid of The Children's Trust. We agreed to start work on the book in June, and to keep meeting weekly until it was completed. Things were moving forward!

In April I went back to Bournemouth Hospital, to find out what was causing my nose and throat problem. I was told that unfortunately there was no specific cause, that I had a case of allergic rhinitis which I was probably going to be stuck with. The catarrh in my ears and throat was really uncomfortable and I was disconcerted to hear that nothing could be done, although the problem could be controlled to some extent with tablets and a nasal spray.

In May, I organised a Tennis Tournament in aid of The Children's Trust. My friend and neighbour Michael Hack set up the competition with the head coach at Christchurch Tennis Facility, Rachel Lambon, and hosted the event with her. (I am indebted to Michael, incidentally, for all his hard work overseeing my events, including the popular Quiz nights).

My business, Purewell Signwriters, sponsored the trophies and supplied banners and flyers to advertise the event. We had Anton's Euro Hoopla Castle, a raffle tombola, cake stand and so on. The weather was good and everyone played brilliant tennis and had a great day out – even Tadworth the Hound showed up. We raised a lot of money, which was divided between the Trust and the tennis club. It all went so well that before the end of the day we booked another event for the same time the following year!

2012 was a big year for the nation. It was the Queen's

Diamond Jubilee, and in June there was a Thames Pageant to celebrate, involving 670 boats. Thousands of spectators lined the banks of the river, and millions more watched on their televisions across the world. It was an amazing spectacle, despite the dreadful weather.

The only thing I was not impressed by was the Royal Barge, which I thought should have been painted in Union Jack colours! But Queen Elizabeth and Prince Philip made me truly proud to be British – standing stoically, smiling and waving in the lashing wind and rain.

Later that month, the shoemaker from Moore Bros. Surgical Shoes said that he would make me some waterproof shoes. I had to pay privately for them, and I also had to agree that he would not be responsible for any injuries caused by me wearing them in the shower. His solution was simple – he adapted a pair of plastic Crocs and they worked a treat. I am reliably informed by friends and family that I no longer smell, which is definitely a good result!

In November I organised another event with the help of Michael Hack. Michael hosted The Children's Trust Charity Ball, to be held at the Menzies Carlton Hotel in Bournemouth. The event started at 7pm and finished late, and it comprised a Bucks Fizz reception, a three course meal, entertainment and dancing and a charity raffle and tombola. Again, I sponsored the posters and tickets.

I was really looking forward to the evening, but I had a nasty fall which meant that I could not attend. I phoned SJ at the Trust to apologise. Fortunately she understood, and the event was very successful in my absence. I had hurt my hip and knee, but luckily I made a rapid recovery and was soon back to normal.

Christmas was approaching. This year we decided to have a small party before Christmas Day, and I invited my friend and her two sons. We had a wonderful time.

Christmas Day was spent as usual. Merry Christmas to everyone who knows us!

Chapter Thirty-One
And Finally

Well, my story is drawing to a close, for now. I am still actively working with The Children's Trust and am very grateful to them for giving me the opportunity to help raise funds for their very worthwhile cause. I am still ticking along with my signwriting business too. And who knows – maybe a new career beckons, as a writer?!

I still suffer pain on a continuous basis, but despite this I greatly enjoy my life. I find that nowadays there is more public awareness of the various issues around disability and people are less likely to stare, or to bully and harass me.

Things have also improved as more legal provision has been made for the disabled, entitling me to help from the State with, for example, a ramp into the house, a special wet room and a stair lift.

The final thing I would like to say is that when my life comes to an end, I would like to be buried in the sea with the fish. After all, I have always been a little shrimp!

The End

Postscript
Morquio's Syndrome

Morquio's Syndrome is a rare genetic disorder. There are a variety of symptoms, including heart and joint problems and below average height. Patients with Morquio's often appear healthy at birth, and the problem is usually diagnosed at between one and three years of age.

Morquio's is caused by a deficiency of specific enzymes, and there is presently no cure. However, clinical trials are currently investigating enzyme replacement therapy, which may slow the progression of the symptoms.

Thank you for buying this book. Please continue to support the causes of the Great Ormond Street Hospital and The Children's Trust. These charities work tirelessly towards the treatment and care of disabled children, and there can be no more worthy cause.

17008681R10221

Printed in Poland
by Amazon Fulfillment
Poland Sp. z o.o., Wrocław